Grasping the Donkey's Tail

UNRAVELING MYSTERIES *from the* CLASSICS *of* ORIENTAL MEDICINE

Peter Eckman

Foreword by Charles Buck

SINGING DRAGON
LONDON AND PHILADELPHIA

First published in 2017
by Singing Dragon
an imprint of Jessica Kingsley Publishers
73 Collier Street
London N1 9BE, UK
and
400 Market Street, Suite 400
Philadelphia, PA 19106, USA

www.singingdragon.com

Front cover image by Neal White.

Library of Congress Cataloging in Publication Data
Title: Grasping the donkey's tail : unraveling mysteries from the classics of oriental medicine / Peter Eckman ; foreword by Charles Buck.
Description: London ; Philadelphia : Jessica Kingsley Publishers, 2017. | Includes bibliographical references.
Identifiers: LCCN 2016051842 (print) | LCCN 2016052662 (ebook) | ISBN 9781848193512 (alk. paper) | ISBN 9780857013101 (ebook)
Subjects: | MESH: Laozi. Dao de jing. | Bianque, active approximately 255 B.C. Nan jing. | Yi jing. | Huainan zi. | Huangdi nei jing. | Medicine, Chinese Traditional--methods | Manuscripts, Medical | Incunabula as Topic
Classification: LCC R601 (print) | LCC R601 (ebook) | NLM WZ 294 | DDC 610.951--dc23

British Library Cataloguing in Publication Data
A CIP catalogue record for this book is available from the British Library

ISBN 978 1 84819 351 2
eISBN 978 0 85701 310 1

Printed and bound in the United States

"Peter Eckman has contributed a number of important ideas and publications to the field of East Asian medicine. Traditional East Asian medicine is founded on principles written down some 2,000 years ago. These canons were seen as somewhat divinely inspired, but in contrast to Western tradition this did not make the authors (known or unknown) or texts inviolable; generations of scholar-practitioners have continued to build on these foundations, and Peter Eckman's eclectic explorations, and most importantly their clinical applications, have contributed greatly to this ongoing process of synthesis, serving to further what Joseph Needham called a confluence of East Asian and modern Western science."

—Andrew Prescott, Former Clinic Director at Jung Tao School of Classical Chinese Medicine

"What has struck me for a long time about Peter Eckman is his insatiable curiosity for his work, in particular Chinese medicine, which reflects in his research and knowledge. In addition, his wide perspective allows him to connect acupuncture with the traditional Chinese sources (Yijing, Taoism) and to unravel them within clinical practice. Thank you for this fundamental work."

—Jean-Marc Kespi, Président d'honneur de l'Association Française d'Acupuncture

Grasping the Donkey's Tail

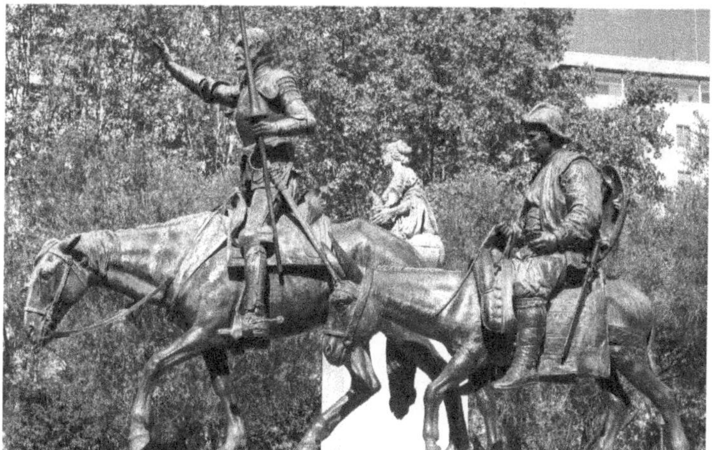

Source: Nicole Ciscato

by the same author

The Compleat Acupuncturist
A Guide to Constitutional and Conditional Pulse Diagnosis
Peter Eckman
Foreword by William Morris
ISBN 978 1 84819 198 3
eISBN 978 0 85701 152 7

of related interest

The Essential Teachings of Sasang Medicine
An Annotated Translation of Lee Je-ma's Dongeui Susei Bowon
Gary Wagman
ISBN 978 1 84819 317 8
eISBN 978 0 85701 270 8

Acupuncture and Chinese Medicine
Roots of Modern Practice
Charles Buck
ISBN 978 1 84819 159 4
eISBN 978 0 85701 133 6

Dedicated to Bian Que
(Circa 5th century BCE)

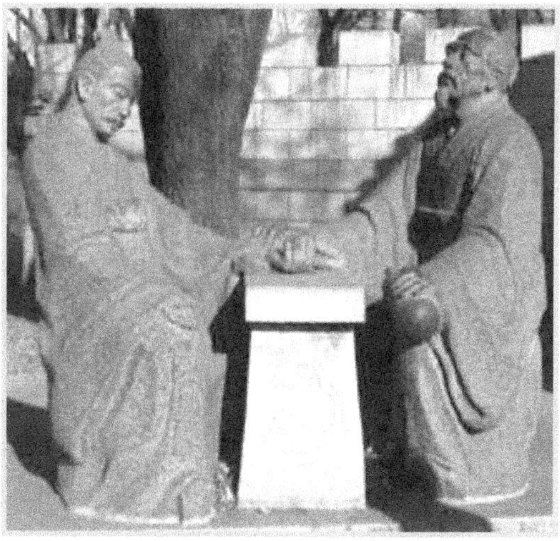

Said to be the first Chinese physician to rely primarily on pulse and physical examination for the diagnosis of disease

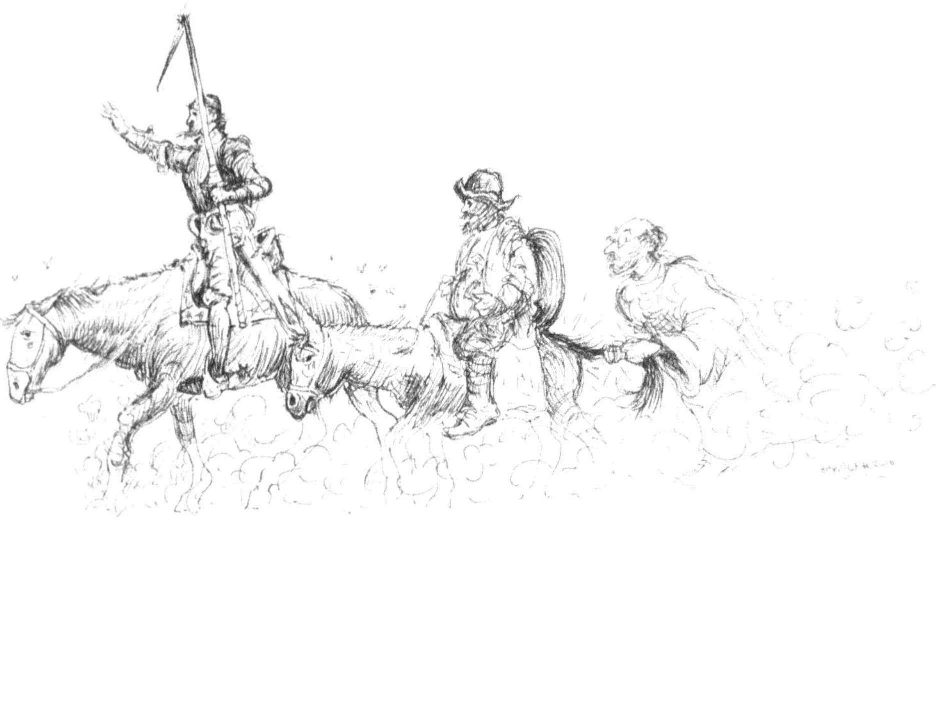

CONTENTS

FOREWORD

I am honoured to have this opportunity to introduce a text by a true pioneer of acupuncture study in the Western world, a man whose work in this field stretches right back to the early 1970s. Happenstance led a few of us onto this path in our youth with the result that we are now living fossils with the insights of this medicine etched into our remains. Our generation was fortunate to be able to access the wisdom of East Asian culture with an ease that was unavailable to previous generations; these opportunities came from advances in Sinology scholarship and the generosity of those born into East Asian culture who made their knowledge available. The scarcity of this knowledge enhanced our perception of its value, it stoked the fires of discovery and helped us to see the subject as precious and worthy of our close attention. We wanted to get to the bottom of it all. Today, with so much more information available, there is a risk we may lose that joy of discovery and the attention we give this subject may become more perfunctory. "Admiring flowers whilst on horseback," as the Chinese idiom has it. So, the scholarship we see in Eckman's *Grasping the Donkey's Tail* is a reminder of our ongoing need to engage in close critical appraisal of this medicine. With luck this work might also help counter the tendency to imagine that we might improve something before we have fully understood it.

The changes we have already witnessed in East–West understanding have been remarkable. We can gauge this by turning our minds back to the zeitgeist of just four decades ago, when China barely existed on our world map and when the word "acupuncture" tinkled almost inaudible amid the other cultural noise of that time. My own pivotal moment came as an undergraduate physiologist in 1976 when, after asking a medical school professor what he considered to be the cutting edge area in neuro-physiology research, he puffed on his pipe and answered, "Oh, acupuncture…definitely!" Although I was somewhat familiar with yin yang, the *Yi Jing* and *Lao Zi*, I had little sense of what acupuncture meant, and was mystified by his words. Only later, after investigating the subject, did I realize that Dr. Purves had followed the acupuncture research in the early 1970s that led to the discovery of the endorphins. Columbus-like, some of us set off with a destination in mind, but then got lost, only to find ourselves somewhere more interesting! Accidental pioneers, we had stumbled through a tiny worm-hole that led us into the vast world of—call it what you will—acupuncture, classical Chinese medicine, Oriental medicine, traditional East Asian medicine, TCM.

The ignorance of that time extended far beyond just acupuncture and Chinese medicine. It's easy to forget that Chinese culture was represented to us back then in a cartoon-like manner, through Kung Fu and Charlie Chan movies garnished with a sprig of *The Reds are Coming!* political propaganda. China was then about as distant from our lives as the planet Mars is today, its language and ideas almost as alien to us as Martian poetry. Apart from Richard Nixon, almost nobody from the West whom we knew had ever actually been there. If you are also a fossil, you perhaps dabbled in the counter-culture of the time, and you may have explored *Lao Zi* and the *Yi Jing* in a naïve way, only to have it later mature into a truer understanding. If this is the case, you will very likely have a good idea of what it takes to reach the level of exploration seen in this book. If instead you are a fresh young thing, I hope you can stretch your mind to appreciate the hard-won insights that lie behind the writing of this book, and that you will aspire to the author's mastery yourself.

Peter Eckman's first encounter with this medicine was in 1973 when he was appointed staff physician at a Los Angeles acupuncture clinic that was run by Korean practitioners. Open to possibilities and open enough to spend time, effort and cash in ongoing study, Peter came to Britain to learn Jack R. Worsley's acupuncture style in 1974. Peter enjoyed a good rapport with his mentor, and on one occasion JR gave him an acupuncture treatment before they headed off to the pub for a beer—directly contradicting a previous JR lecture on the prohibition of combining alcohol with acupuncture! This is a lesson in learning from one's own experience and never taking words or teachers as infallible providers of absolute truth. This close relationship with Worsley in those early days meant that Peter was especially well placed to publish his 1996 book, *In the Footsteps of the Yellow Emperor: Tracing the History of Traditional Acupuncture*, which detailed his quest to find the origins of JR's Five Element style of practice.

When we read *Grasping the Donkey's Tail*, Peter Eckman's continual hunger for additional perspectives is evident, a quest that led him to study with the founding father of ear acupuncture (Dr. Paul Nogier), and also with numerous renowned Japanese, Vietnamese, Chinese and Taiwanese masters, with French-Vietnamese style acupuncture experts, and more recently with the US-based Daoist lineage master Jeffery Yuen, but especially with the lineage originators of two Korean styles of acupuncture. Evident too is the way he has worked hard to make sense of the abstruse texts that founded classical acupuncture. Eckman has delved into the puzzle of the often-obscure meanings of the words, chapters and verses of these classical texts. With the interested and investigative mind of a true physician he has sought to reconcile his historical explorations with real clinical practice. Clearly he knows that written knowledge has limited value—its worth lies more in creating a state of readiness for the practical wisdom that is to be gained through actual clinical application. With minds that are suitably primed we can realize the truths inherent in this medicine—clinical mastery is the accumulation of moments of insight that happen in the course of our encounters with patients. This realization, that theory and reality intertwine, and that reality normally trumps theory, is a hallmark of greatness that we see throughout Chinese medicine's history. Great physicians are pragmatists whose theories are tested by their clinical work. This you will see in Eckman's writing.

What is presented here is not a comprehensive survey of classical medicine. Indeed, it cannot be so because to faithfully and fully represent the minds of Han dynasty China's scholars turns out to be a near-impossible challenge. Instead, you will get the author's insights on some aspects of Daoist styles of acupuncture and more specifically on the subject of pulse diagnosis. The book opens with Eckman's perspectives on *Yi Jing* study that are a cornerstone of classical acupuncture and that are also fundamental to Korean constitutional acupuncture (a subject that was detailed in his previous text for Singing Dragon, *The Compleat Acupuncturist*). After this he examines issues of cognition and spirit from the *Lao Zi*, before coming to grips with a crucial idea needed to understand Han dynasty Chinese medicine thinking—the ancient concept of Gan Ying (感应, resonant causality). Gan Ying conceptualizes the ways that things in nature mutually respond to each other, and the ways that influence and change operate. This is important because, at its heart, Daoist medicine is about understanding the mechanisms of change and transformation in the natural environment and in people. In a tour-de-force, Peter Eckman guides us through the main early text on this subject, namely Chapter 6 of the western Han dynasty classic the *Huai Nan Zi*.

Moving on then to pulse diagnosis, Eckman examines this subject from the perspective of the foundational medical classics the *Su Wen*, *Ling Shu* and *Nan Jing* (Plain Questions, Miraculous Pivot and Difficult Classic). We benefit from his detailed study of the original texts to get to the intent of the original authors. Included in this section is an appraisal of the neglected subject of the examination of the carotid artery pulse, and its relationship to the radial artery pulse. We also learn the experiences of the modern masters that Peter has studied with, plus conclusions based on his application of these approaches clinically. His critical appraisal of the pulse discussions in the *Nan Jing* brings new clarity to their application in constitutional acupuncture. Peter then clears a track for us to wander through Wang Shu-he's (1997) *Mai Jing* (Pulse Classic), helping to resolve some of the conflicting interpretations of this key text.

Peter Eckman and I share a similar mind-set, we have a fascination with the treasure that is to be found in the book's subject, and our careers in this medicine have many parallels. I believe that we share a conviction that the classical tradition sought to promote rational and practical medicine rooted in careful study and reflection, and that the task of a physician is to develop understanding by combining personal cultivation with critical reflection. I admire the extent to which Peter Eckman has achieved this.

Besides its academic and practical value, this book also embodies the growing realisation that the adage "information is power" no longer quite holds true today. It used to be that the people who had the information held the power; but now that information is cheap and easily available, almost everyone has access to almost everything. The problem now is not that we do not have the information, it is that we have a bewildering excess of the stuff, so power now lies more in the hands of those who have the ability to navigate meaningfully through this information and guide others through the maze. Nowhere is this special skill more desperately needed than in our field. I see Peter Eckman as a fellow traveller and a true pioneer in this medicine who is especially well placed to guide us and share his own hard-won insights with others, and who does this with clarity and charm.

Charles Buck
Past Chairman of the British Acupuncture Council
Chester UK, September 2016

ACKNOWLEDGMENTS

I must start out by expressing my gratitude towards Olga Fedina, Hector Moret and John Maher who hosted my seminar in Barcelona and showed me an insider's view of Spain. Without that beginning, my fateful encounter with Cervantes' characters wouldn't have occurred, and this book might still be gestating.

Next I must thank Charles Buck for contributing the Foreword. We first met at the annual symposium of the British Acupuncture Council a few years ago as co-presenters, and immediately recognized kindred spirits in each other, having traversed more or less the same professional path on opposite sides of the pond.

Once again I am fortunate to have the encouragement and artistic contributions of Neal White, who has put his pen and ink imprimatur on virtually everything I have written since I began as the official book reviewer for the *Journal of Traditional Acupuncture* back in 1991, now sadly defunct lo these many years. Igor Simonov was very generous in granting me permission to share aspects of his research that he has not yet published himself. Ian Harp enthusiastically shared his experiences in applying classical dogma in clinical practice.

Several of my peers have read the initial draft of this work, and provided invaluable feedback, catching more faux pas than I would like to admit. Special thanks to Andrew Prescott and Leo

Lok in that regard, who also provoked me to think more deeply about the interpretations of the classical texts to be found herein. And of course, my publisher, without whose belief in the value of my work, you would not be reading this. None of us stands alone, so I thank all of my predecessors, teachers, colleagues, students and patients.

Last, but not least, a big *spasibo* to my wife Marina Chentsova, whose photographical whimsy you are sure to encounter if you get to the finish line. May you enjoy reading this as much as I enjoyed the writing of it. Correspondence is always welcome at healingmountain@aol.com (just include "acupuncture" in the subject line, or risk consignment to the spam file).

PREFACE

Why such a preposterous title? I had recently finished teaching a seminar in Barcelona, after which my wife and I spent some time exploring the wonders of Spain, when I found myself in Madrid, gazing at the imposing statue of Don Quixote and his squire, Sancho Panza, in the Plaza de España. The next thing I knew, I had to grab that donkey's tail, because something was missing: The Don, high on his horse, head in the clouds, reminded me of Heaven, that idealized place of perfection; Sancho, plodding along behind on his poor donkey, reminded me of Earth, the reality we all deal with on a daily basis, if we manage to keep our sanity; but something was missing. Man, in Oriental medicine, is the mediator between the ethereal and the material worlds, and provides for the possibility of conscious understanding of the other two realms, but only by being in touch with them. My seminar, being on pulse diagnosis, had inspired me to explore some insights that seemed to spring from the experience of using touch as my primary check on reality, and so, following Heaven and Earth, I grabbed the donkey's tail.

If you don't care for that explanation, perhaps you'd be happier knowing that I'm an insufferable punster, who couldn't pass up the opportunity of conflating Don Quixote and donkey. Don't say I didn't warn you.

Introduction

To know that you are ignorant is best,
To know what you do not, is a disease.

LAO ZI, CHAPTER 71[1]

This book is about acupuncture and is written for acupuncturists, but there is nothing to stop an interested layperson from acquiring some familiarity with the mysteries I discuss. The treatise examines a series of passages from various Chinese classics, whose conventional interpretation left me puzzled. Based on my many years of practice, together with my meager skills at reading classical Chinese, I have come to my own conclusions about the meaning of these texts, and my interpretations form the content of this treatise. Had these been mere speculative interpretations, I would not consider them worth publishing, but I have actually found them to be invaluable guides to more effective acupuncture treatments. At first I considered calling this book *The Difficulties of the Difficulties* because it deals (among other material) with some of the obscure passages in *The Yellow Emperor's Inner Classic* (*Nei Jing*), as does (according to many authorities) the *Classic of Difficulties* (*Nan Jing*), but my proposed title sounded a bit too esoteric even to me. Another famous text, *Correcting the Errors*

1 Blakney (1980) *The Sayings of Lao Zi*, p.142. 知不知上; 不知知病.

in the Forest of Medicine (*Yi Lin Gai Cuo*) by Wang Qing-ren, had already covered exactly the kind of treatise I had decided to write, so that title was already taken. In the end, I decided on the title you see, which, though playful, is also meant to convey my most serious and pragmatic thoughts about the practice of acupuncture.

We live in an age that has become more and more materialistic. Since the industrial revolution, science has gradually replaced religion as the primary orientation in most civilized societies. Nowhere is this more evident than in the field of medicine, where "evidence-based research" has become the gold standard for sanctioned practices by governments and professional associations alike. This trend has gone so far that the practice of medicine is adjudged to be either scientific or not, based on its acceptance of evidence-based criteria. Even in the field of Chinese medicine, as codified by the Chinese government under the rubric of TCM (Traditional Chinese Medicine), the thrust has been to discard any of its traditional aspects that do not stand up to modern scientific scrutiny.[2]

I believe the pendulum has swung too far in the direction of materialist reductionism. While I am all for the benefits

2 Paul Unschuld, in his *Journal of Chinese Medicine* interview (Rosenberg 2013, p.4), reported the following: "Outright condemnations of Chinese medicine by the political leadership ended after the founding of the People's Republic of China, but the hidden agenda has remained the same. A committee was ordered in the early 1950s until the mid-1960s to define those elements of Chinese historical medicine that might be worth continuing in a new China devoted to Marxism–Maoism as its social science, and Western science as its natural science. This committee created 'Traditional Chinese Medicine'... The bottom-line has been to slowly decrease the impact of ancient theory, and to use modern Western scientific approaches to research...in a modern biomedical environment... Hence in 2007, the Chinese authorities invited ministers of science and ministers of health of 50 leading nations to China to resolve a Beijing Declaration of TCM. Its main message was twofold. First, 'TCM is part of modern biomedicine', and second 'The basis of TCM is molecular biology'."

that science has provided for humankind, we are also seeing a tremendous cost in terms of the side effects of pollution, global warming, and other ecological challenges. Western medicine has also introduced a plethora of iatrogenic diseases and morbidities caused by the side effects of its powerful pharmaceuticals. Being a Western medical doctor and also a Ph.D. in physiology, I feel qualified to make these assertions without coming across as a new-age ideologue. The problem with Western medicine, as I see it, is that it has lost its awareness that there is a part of being human that is beyond the mere physical body. I choose to call this missing part our spirit, which while intangible, is what animates our lives and then is absent from our bodies when our lives are over.

So, what is the answer to this dichotomy between religion and science, spirit and matter? I believe the answer lies in re-examining our basic assumptions about what we really mean by the term "science," and in doing so I think we might recover the tremendous scientific achievements made by past cultures that did not exclude the spiritual nature of human existence from their view of "science." In my more than 40 years of study and practice of Oriental medicine, I have discovered that its classical texts proposed a synthesis of these two poles of the nature of reality, spirit and matter, and that from ancient times there was always a thread of scientific thinking present, admittedly intermixed with the kind of irrational beliefs that proliferated in those societies.

My purpose then, in writing this book, is to examine what I believe to be some crucial passages from the classical Chinese texts that can help guide us to a better understanding of ourselves and the potential of Oriental medical science to benefit humankind. To me, science is essentially a commitment to a careful examination of reality, with the aim of being able to thereby accurately predict future observations. Joseph Needham (1956, pp.73 and 286) and others after him were adamant about how meticulous the ancient Chinese were in observing every aspect of nature, and in proposing various theories to account for them as a basis for predicting future outcomes. I see this as scientific investigation. I will examine how this kind of scientific investigation has provided guidelines for the effective use of acupuncture, my specialty, which can be built upon by today's practitioners. This Eastern branch of science is inductive, qualitative and synthetic, as opposed to the deductive, quantitative and analytic nature of Western science—neither is superior to nor more correct than the other. They are simply different ways of organizing information about the natural world.

The ideas in this treatise are my own (unless stipulated otherwise), and of course other practitioners are free to disagree with any of my assertions, but having been a successful acupuncturist for over 40 years leads me to believe that there is great wisdom still buried in the ancient texts, which can be resurrected for a more comprehensive and more efficacious practice of medicine in these modern times.

Chapter 1

Yì Jīng 易經

THE CLASSIC OF CHANGES

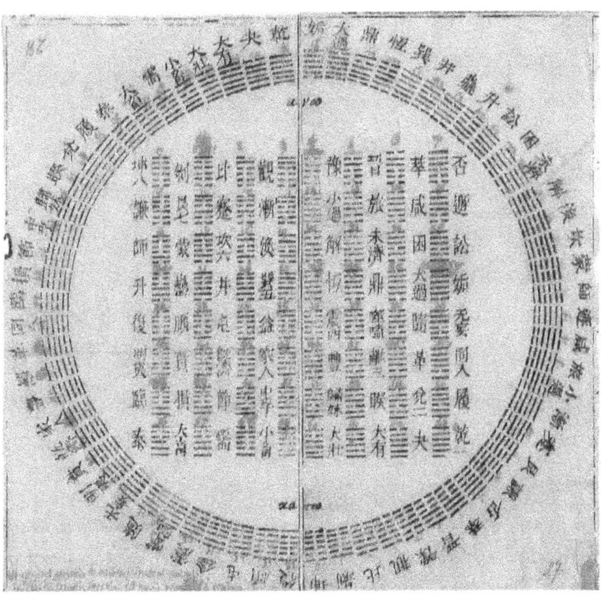

Figure 1.1 Diagram of *Yi Jing* hexagrams owned by Gottfried Wilhelm Leibniz, 1701[1]

Source: commons.wikimedia.org

1 This diagram was sent to the mathematician Leibniz (co-inventor of calculus) by the French Jesuit Joachim Bouvet. The Arabic numerals written on the diagram were added by Leibniz.

The *Yi Jing* is historically one of China's oldest books. While it is not ordinarily considered to be a medical text, throughout the ages many commentators on Oriental medicine have seen in it the inspiration for much of Oriental medicine's subsequent development.[2] In the West, however, this book is primarily treated as a somewhat magical guide to divinatory practices. In the introduction to his highly respected translation of the *Yi Jing*, Richard Wilhelm noted that early on, Wang Pi, in the 3rd century, "wrote about the meaning of the Book of Changes as a book of wisdom, not as a book of divination" (Wilhelm and Baynes 1977, p.lx) and commented that it was the root of both Confucianism and Daoism (ibid., p.xlvii), each of which made significant contributions to the development of Oriental medicine. erhaps the most perceptive comment that Wilhelm made was that the eight trigrams, which are fundamental components of the classical text, formed families of "father, mother, three sons and three daughters, not in the mythological sense in which the Greek gods peopled Olympus, but in what might be called an abstract sense, that is, they represented not objective entities but functions" (ibid., p.l). This sentence can be used to characterize the essential difference between Western

2 See *The Book of Changes in Traditional Oriental Medicine* by this author for a detailed examination of how the *Yi Jing* underlies almost all the theoretical concepts in Oriental medicine (Eckman 1988). More recently, Alex Scrimgeour (2011) cited the following quotations from eminent Chinese physicians in his Bac. Dissertation on the *Yi Jing* and Chinese Medicine: 醫者易也, "*Yī zhě yì yě*—Real medicine is thoroughly based on *Yi Jing* science" (Zhāng Jièbīn), and "Medicine cannot be mastered until you have studied the *Yi Jing*" (Sun Si Miao). Lorraine Wilcox (2016) has translated other quotes from Zhāng Jièbīn: 醫易同原, "Medicine and the Changes have the same source," and 雖陰陽已備於（內經），而變 化莫大乎 （周易）, "Although *Nèi Jīng* already possesses *yīn-yáng*, nothing is better for [understanding its] mutations and transformations than the *Zhōu Yì*." *Zhou Yi* was the name of the *Yi Jing* prior to its addition of the commentaries known as the ten wings.

and Eastern modes of approaching medicine: the former from a structural viewpoint and the latter from a functional one. The famous psychoanalyst Carl Jung wrote the Foreword to Wilhelm's translation, and succinctly captured how this difference in viewpoint leads to a difference in attitude towards the practice of medicine by stating "nowhere else do we become more accustomed to adopting methods that work even though for a long time we may not know why they work. Unexpected cures may arise from questionable therapies and unexpected failures from allegedly reliable methods" (ibid., p.xxxiv). Close to 100 percent of my patients would identify that quotation as expressing the reason they have chosen acupuncture rather than pharmaceutical medicine to address their health concerns.

I chose the *Yi Jing* as the focus of Chapter 1 specifically because I see it as the fountainhead that led to the differing medical traditions in China and Korea,[3] a subject that has led to some confusion arising from terminological ambiguity. The structure of the *Yi Jing* is based on solid and broken lines, commonly referred to as yáng and yīn respectively.[4] As single lines these would be called monograms, as pairs of lines they are bigrams, as triplets they are referred to as trigrams, and as sextuplets they are known as the more familiar hexagrams. The trigrams form a very

3 The unique approaches developed in Korea and China illustrate one of the reasons I have been using Oriental medicine rather than Chinese medicine to denote the generic group of practices I wish to contrast with Western medicine.

4 The oldest parts of the *Yi Jing* don't actually mention the terms yin and yang. Instead they refer to "yielding" and "solid." Yin and yang make their first appearance there in Section 1 of the *Great Commentary*, one of the later "wings" or appendices of the *Yi Jing*, in Chapter 5, "One yin, one yang is called the Dao: 一陰一陽之謂道." Chapter 11 states, "Therefore the Yi incorporates the Great Axis (Tai Ji) which produces the two primal forces. The two primal forces produce four images (xiang). The four images produce the eight trigrams: 易有太極, 是生兩儀, 兩儀生四象, 四象生八卦." Translation of *Yi Jing* by Wu (1991, pp.266 and 271).

important conceptual basis for two of the most characteristic theoretical concepts in Chinese medicine: the Five Elements doctrine and the Three Yin/Three Yang doctrine, each of which informs much of acupunctural and herbal medical theory and practice.[5] The bigrams, on the other hand, more commonly and literally translated as the Four Images (四象 *sì xiàng* in Chinese and *sa sang* in Korean) were chosen as the fundamental theoretical concept in many styles of Korean acupuncture and herbal medicine. The reason for confusion is that some of the same words are used to name the acupuncture meridians and the images (bigrams), but the meanings denoted are different in these two cases:

> The Four Images are 太陽 Tài Yáng (Taeyang), 太陰 Tài Yīn (Taeum), 少陽 Shǎo Yáng (Soyang) and 少陰 Shǎo Yīn (Soeum) to give both their Chinese and Korean names. This grouping of four terms is the basis of both Sa Sang herbal medicine, and of several variants of Korean acupuncture, including Tae Guk (太極, Tài Jí in Chinese) Acupuncture and Korean Constitutional Acupuncture.[6] Had I chosen to

5 Eckman (1988) *The Book of Changes in Traditional Oriental Medicine.* There is much controversy about the translation of the Chinese term 五行 wǔxíng into English. As with many Chinese terms, there is no single definitive translation that covers all the connotations of wǔ xíng. Five Elements was the first to become popular in Western languages, thanks to the influential work of Soulié de Morant, and I have kept it because of its historical precedence and common usage. The style of acupuncture based on this doctrine, exemplified by the teachings of J.R. Worsley, retains this terminology of Five Elements, while practitioners of most other styles of acupuncture prefer alternative terms such as Five Phases or Five Movements, terms that are also preferred by most scholarly writers. I think all of these choices are acceptable, as long as the user realizes that each one captures only part of the multiple meanings conveyed by this important Chinese term.

6 These methodologies are discussed in some detail in the author's publication *The Compleat Acupuncturist* (Eckman 2014).

> use only the Chinese characters for these terms, rather than their Romanized alphabetical names, there would have been no difference between the Korean and Chinese nomenclature; however, one significant feature of languages based on Chinese characters is that each character can have multiple meanings, and the appropriate one to choose is often governed by the context in which it is used. When discussing the Four Images, I prefer to translate them as Old Yang, Old Yin, Young Yang and Young Yin respectively.[7] On the other hand, when discussing the Three Yin/Three Yang nomenclature, I translate these very same characters as Greater Yang, Greater Yin, Lesser Yang and Lesser Yin respectively. The two missing terms in meridian nomenclature are Fading Yin (厥陰 Jué Yīn) and Bright Yang (陽明 Yáng Míng).

To illustrate the confusion that frequently arises, let us examine Tai Yang in both contexts. In Sa Sang usage, Tai Yang refers to a strong Lung together with a weak Liver conformation, while in the Three Yin/Three Yang usage, Tai Yang refers to the Meridians and their associated Fǔ Organs consisting of the Urinary Bladder and the Small Intestine. Obviously, without knowing the context, these terms can lead to a complete misunderstanding in using either written or spoken words. In order to minimize confusion, I present both systems in Table 1.1, using the standard Chinese terminology. In keeping with this book's theme of touch,

7 Stephen Boyanton posted the following comment on Facebook Scholars of Chinese Medicine 8/7/16: "Dating of the various parts of the Yi Jing is tricky, but the 'four images (sixiang 四象)' appear at least as early as the Xici 繫辭 section of the text referred to as shaoyang 少陽, laoyang 老陽, shaoyin 少陰 and laoyin 老陰." As lao unambiguously means "old," my choice of young and old here has scholarly support.

I want to point out that both Sa Sang diagnosis and Three Yang/Three Yin diagnosis are best identified via pulse examination.[8]

TABLE 1.1 COMPARISON OF FOUR-FOLD AND SIX-FOLD TERMINOLOGIES

Four Images/Sì Xiàng (Sa Sang) theory

Tai Yang	Strong Lung	Weak Liver
Tai Yin	Strong Liver	Weak Lung
Shao Yang	Strong Spleen	Weak Kidney
Shao Yin	Strong Kidney	Weak Spleen

Three Yang/Three Yin theory

Tai Yang	Urinary Bladder	Small Intestine
Yang Ming	Stomach	Large Intestine
Shao Yang	Gall Bladder	Triple Heater
Tai Yin	Spleen/Pancreas	Lung
Shao Yin	Kidney	Heart
Jue Yin	Liver	Pericardium

Most readers are more likely to be familiar with the Chinese, rather than the Korean, usages of these four terms in reference to Meridians and Organ systems. Thus, I would like to say a few words about the Korean Sa Sang approach, which are not detailed as such in any of its texts (to the best of my knowledge), but which I've developed to clarify this confusing terminology for those previously familiar only with the Chinese applications. What I will present is an allegorical interpretation of the usage of these four terms to represent the development of mental,

8 The pulse diagnostic methodology of both Sa Sang medicine and Korean Constitutional Acupuncture (based on Sa Sang theory) are explained in *The Compleat Acupuncturist*. One method of Three Yang/Three Yin pulse diagnosis is also introduced in that text, but a more comprehensive and probably earlier method is discussed in Chapter 5 of the present text.

emotional, and spiritual growth, which were important guiding concepts in the Confucian ideology that Lee (whose work was published in the late 1800s, and translated into English in 1966) used in his writing about Sa Sang theory. Although each of us has a constitutional relationship to one of the Four Image (Sa Sang) types, we all have the same possibility of developing our higher faculties through the same four stages, as in the following explanation.

Sa Sang medicine is based on the idea that there are four jiāo 焦, rather than the three of Chinese medicine.[9] They are pictured in Figure 1.2 as Lower, Lower Middle, Upper Middle and Upper jiāo, corresponding respectively to Kidney, Liver, Spleen and Lung. Roughly these correspond to the physical placement of the familiar anatomical structures associated with these names, but the placement of the two parts of the Middle jiāo are debatable even in the Chinese three-jiāo tradition. This difference of opinion explains why in Chinese medicine the Liver is sometimes associated with the Lower jiāo while the Spleen is always associated with the Middle jiāo.

If we think of the jiāo as potentially representing something like the Chakras of Ayurveda, there is a sense in which we start our lives centered in, and from, the first Chakra, and gradually work our spiritual development upwards (from Earth to Heaven). The lower jiāo is like the first Chakra, concerned with survival issues, and it resonates with the Kidney (fear, caution, the

9 The ideal translation and meaning of the term jiāo 焦 is controversial. It is frequently rendered as "warmer," "heater," or "burner." I have found in my clinical practice that individuals whose constitutions are either Young Yin or Young Yang frequently are distinctly colder in the lower jiāo, whereas those whose constitutions are either Old Yin or Old Yang are distinctly colder in the lower middle jiāo (see Figure 1.2). This is not only a useful diagnostic indicator, but serves to reinforce my contention that Oriental medicine's theories are derived from "reality-based" observations, and merit classification as a branch of science.

unknown) as does the Water Element, with its responsibility for the original qì and the jīng. I call 少陰 in this case Young Yin as my translation of Soeum, and Lee (1966) identified this constitution as having a strong Kidney and a weak Spleen as its defining characteristic. In a circular depiction (Figure 1.3) it is at the bottom (North) because the Kidney is the Foundation and Origin of each individual life. The Kidney's spiritual correlate is the Zhì 志 (will, as in will to life).

Young Yin then evolves to Old Yin 太陰 (Taeum) which manifests constitutionally with a strong Liver and a weak Lung as its defining characteristic. On the circle it is in the East position, which corresponds to the Wood Element. In Chakra terms it is concerned with duality and sexuality (a major issue in planning and decision making), and the exploration of others as distinct from self, but the emphasis is on self more than on others, thus the rebelliousness and impetuosity as we mature from childhood to adolescence. One might say our Hún 魂 runs wild, with no real inherent constraint.

As we mature further, we progress upwards to the Young Yang stage 少陽 (Soyang), which is characterized constitutionally by a strong Spleen and a weak Kidney. Here, the "other" has more emphasis than the self, as we begin to recognize that we are not more important than all the other beings with whom we share resources (the Yì 意 is replacing the Hún 魂 as the spiritual focus). This is at the top of the circle (South), but because there is no Fire Element (which would normally be placed there) in Sa Sang theory, it is now replaced by the Earth Element with its focus on sympathy and empathy.[10] This spiritual progression explains why the Spleen is metaphorically located above the Liver.

10 Kespi (2012) has noted that humans have two centers in acupuncture theory. Fire (the Heart) is the "center-source," while Earth (Spleen/Pancreas-Stomach) is the "center-site."

Finally, we reach the Old Yang stage 太陽 (Taeyang), which is characterized constitutionally by a strong Lung and a weak Liver. Here our consciousness is focused on the highest of the Zang Organs (the Lung), which rules our spiritual aspirations, as in our connection to Heaven, but also our process of letting go of attachment to our material existence (dependent on the Pò 魄), as the circle turns and we find ourselves located in the West. This is the phase of preparation for (physical) death, but also that of (metaphysical) preparation for rebirth.

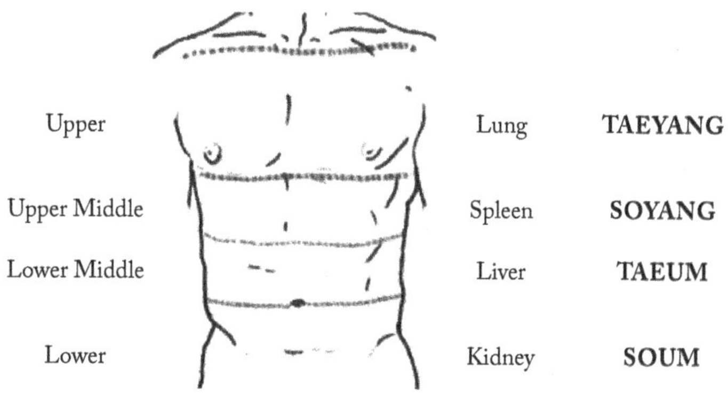

Figure 1.2 The Four Jiao model
Source: Neal White and Peter Eckman

Figure 1.3 shows a graphic representation of the Sa Sang organization, with Young Yin transforming into Old Yin, which transforms into Young Yang, which transforms into Old Yang, ready to start the cycle over again. In the Sa Sang model, as mentioned, the Fire Element is not included, but its position is occupied by the Earth Zàng, the Spleen/Pancreas. Otherwise the Wood Zàng (Liver) is in the East, the Metal Zàng (Lung) is in the West, and the Water Zàng (Kidney) is in the North, as expected. While there is a certain degree of correspondence of the Sa Sang model with many tenets of Chinese medicine, there are also major differences. For example, there is no concept of coupled Zàng and Fǔ Organs or Meridians, the Five Elements are not actually discussed nor applied in diagnosis and treatment, and as originally formulated, Sa Sang medicine was purely a herbal modality, and did not include acupuncture. However, as predicted by its originator, Lee Je-ma (Lee 1966), eventually acupuncture styles based on Sa Sang theory were developed, as mentioned above. In order to apply Sa Sang theory to acupuncture, however, some adjustment was needed to include the Fire Element, with its four Meridians and Organ systems.

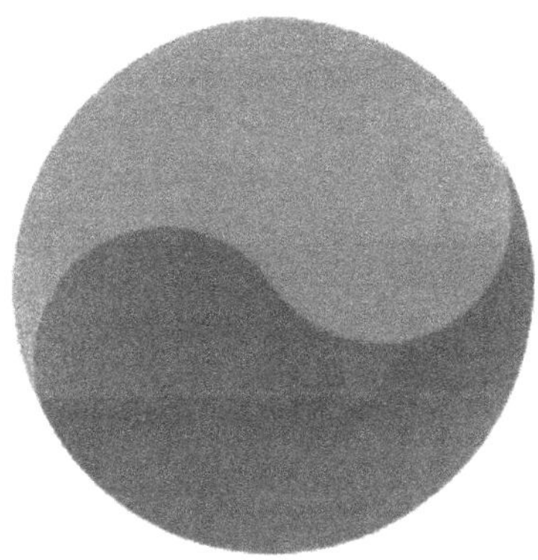
Soyang: SP Excess, KI Deficiency
(HE 3+, KI 3+, SP 3–)
Young Yang
Taeum:
LV Excess,
LU
Deficiency
(HE 4+,
LU 9+,
LV 3–)
Old Yin
Old Yang
Taeyang:
LU Excess,
LV
Deficiency
(He 8+,
LV 3+,
LU 9–)
Young Yin
Soeum: KI Excess, SP Deficiency
(HE 7+, SP 3+, LI 4–)

Figure 1.3 The Sa Sang orientation and treatment points for Tae Guk Acupuncture
Source: Peter Eckman

I have not previously published material on Tae Guk Acupuncture, which was originated by Lee Byeonghaeng in Korea (date unknown). This system found a simple way to begin integrating the Fire Element into an essentially four-part theory based on the other Elements, thereby keeping very close to classical Sa Sang theory. The four Constitutions of that theory were primarily treated by simply tonifying the Source Points of the deficient Meridians and sedating (dispersing) the Source Points of the excessive Meridians, as follows:

> Young Yang (Soyang), which has deficient Kidney and excess Spleen, was treated by tonifying KI 3 and sedating SP 3. Old Yang (Taeyang), which has deficient Liver and excess Lung, was treated by tonifying LV 3 and sedating LU 9. Old Yin (Taeum), which has deficient Lung and excess Liver, was treated by tonifying LU 9 and sedating LV 3. Young Yin (Soeum), which has deficient Spleen and excess Kidney, was treated by tonifying SP 3, but instead of sedating KI 3, Lee Byeonghaeng chose to sedate LI 4, most likely because some schools of Oriental medical thought teach that one should never sedate the Kidney. In Sa Sang theory (which doesn't recognize either the Five Element doctrine, nor the Yin/Yang coupling of Zàng and Fǔ Meridians), the Large Intestine is considered part of the Kidney system, rather than the Lung system, so its Source Point was chosen for sedation in this case. Finally, the Fire Element was incorporated by choosing a point on the Heart Meridian for treatment of each of the constitutions according to the general rule: use either the Element Point corresponding to the deficient Organ of that Constitution, or the corresponding Element Point of the controller of the excess Organ. For Young Yang, HE 3, the Water Point is tonified. This reflects the rule of

> choosing the deficient Organ's Element Point, but also can be viewed as the Point of the Element (Water) that controls Fire, which is normally the Element in the South position in Chinese medicine, but is occupied by the excess Spleen (Earth Element) in Sa Sang dogma. These adjustments show an attempt to integrate the theoretical discrepancies between Korean and Chinese medical theory. The other Constitutions' Point on the Heart Meridian follow the rule of tonifying the Element Point corresponding to the Meridian that controls the Excessive Organ, that is: HE 8 for Old Yang (Fire controls Metal), HE 7 for Young Yin (Earth controls Water) and HE 4 for Old Yin (Metal controls Wood).

Tae Guk Acupuncture never became as widely practiced in Korea as its successor, Korean Constitutional Acupuncture (KCA), first introduced by Kuon Dowon in 1965, which has since spread worldwide. KCA represents a further attempt to integrate Sa Sang and Chinese medical theories, but also introduced some conceptual aspects from the Western medical thinking of Hans Selye, a Nobel Prize nominee. I have described the various iterations of Kuon's methodology previously (Eckman 2014), so I will not go into detail here, but just note some of the highlights. The four Constitutions of Sa Sang medicine were doubled to make eight types, a Chang (Zàng) and a Bu (Fǔ) "temperament" for each of the original four Constitutions. Each of these eight types has a unique "Constitutional Pulse" signature that never changes throughout the life of any given individual. The constitutional acupuncture treatments in KCA were all based on the Four Needle Technique, a Medieval Korean application of Five Element theory. While there still was no Fire Element Constitution, the Fire Element was treated via the first of the Auxiliary Formulas that Kuon introduced, that being the

Neuropsychological Formula. Kuon's thinking was influenced by the *Nan Jing*, and so I will return to some discussion of KCA in Chapter 6, but will explore my current thoughts about it in the Addendum.

Chapter 2

Lǎo Zǐ 老子 *or Dào Dé Jīng* 道德經

THE WAY AND ITS POWER

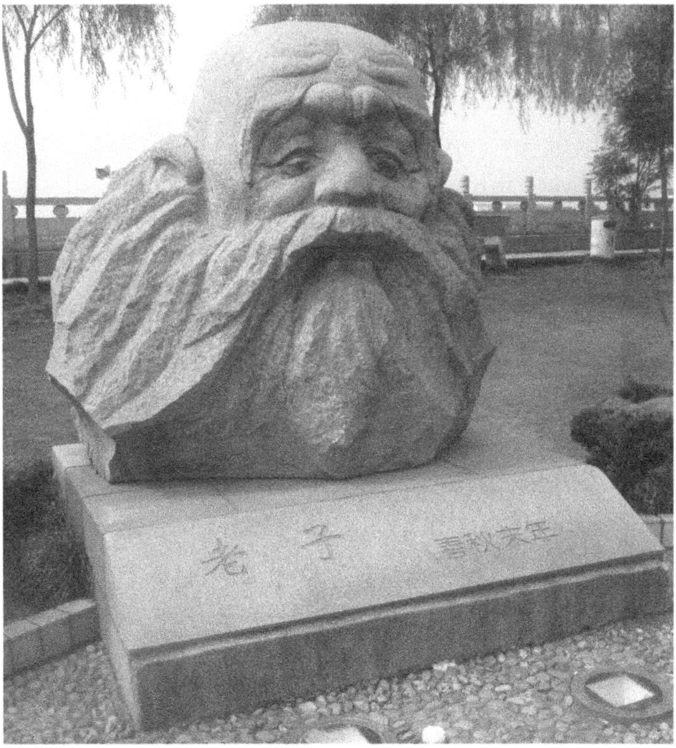

Figure 2.1 The Old Master, Lao Zi
Source: Harold Groven

Daoist philosophy was already mentioned as being rooted in the *Yi Jing*, but its first classical text is attributed to a legendary figure called the "Old Master," about whom no reliable historical data have been documented (Figure 2.1). So, it is fitting that the opening remarks of the text attributed to him seem at first glance to be mystical, to the point of appearing rather useless as a rational guide to something as concrete as the practice of acupuncture: "The Dao that can be trodden is not the enduring and unchanging Dao. The name that can be named is not the enduring and unchanging name."[1] Translations into English often leave Dao in the original Chinese because it can take on so many different meanings, but most often is rendered as "The Way." Literally, that would change the English opening phrase to "The Way that can be Wayed." No wonder it is confusing. These first two sentences are so broad and deep in their meaning that I will not try to fashion a new translation into English; however, I believe that there is a corollary that can be derived from these sentences that is very fitting for understanding my point of view regarding classical texts, and their relationship to scientific inquiry. It is succinctly stated in the common English phrase, "The map is not the territory," an important truth that is characteristic of all sciences, whether Eastern or Western.[2] In acupuncture theory and practice there are many guidelines that have been developed from the classics, or from later works, which should be viewed as embodying the maps and other descriptions we have given to reality, not as reality-in-itself. There will always be some aspects

1 ctext.org/dao-de-jing 道可道, 非常道. 名可名, 非常名.

2 The Chinese text has a much broader set of meanings, but the present discussion is focused on this most practical aspect only. The quoted saying is attributed to Alfred Korzybski (1879–1950), a Polish-American independent scholar who developed a field called general semantics. He first introduced the statement in a meeting of the American Association for the Advancement of Science in New Orleans in 1931.

of nature that can never be fully described because descriptions are like words and maps, while the Dao is nature (or natural law), unfiltered through the lens of human consciousness. This idea is reprised in Chapter 25 thus:

> "Man takes his law from the Earth; the Earth takes its law from Heaven; Heaven takes its law from the Dao. The law of the Dao is its being what it is."[3]

Somewhat later, another Daoist philosopher wrote in the eponymous 莊子 *Zhuāng Zǐ*:

> "This is the Dao… It has Its root and ground (of existence) in Itself. Before there were heaven and earth, from of old, there It was, securely existing. From It came the mysterious existences of spirits, from It the mysterious existence of God. It produced heaven; It produced earth. It was before the Tai-ji."

And:

> "All things are produced from the Earth and return to the Earth. Therefore I will leave you, and enter the gate of the Unending, to enjoy myself in the fields of the Illimitable. I will blend my light with that of the sun and moon, and will endure while heaven and earth endure."[4]

---

3 ctext.org/dao-de-jing 人法地, 地法天, 天法道, 道法自然.

4 *Zhuang Zi* (Outer Chapters) 3 "Letting Be, and Exercising Forbearance" (Legge, J., trans.). He rendered shen gui (spirits-ghosts) as spirits and shen di (spirits-emperor) as God, a rather modern Western interpretation. He left tai ji untranslated, but chose "illimitable" for wu ji. 夫道, … 自本自根, 未有天地, 自古以固存; 神鬼神帝, 生天生地; 在太極之先而不為高, 在六極之下而不為深; 先天地生而不為久上及有虞, 下及五伯; 傅說得之, 以相武丁, 奄有天下. 自本自根, 未有天地, 自古以固存; 神鬼神帝, 生天生地; 在太極之先而不為高. … 今夫百昌, 皆生於土而反於土, 故余將去女, 入無窮之門, 以遊無極之野. 吾與日月參光, 吾與天地為常. http://ctext.org/zhuangzi/letting-be-and-exercising-forbearance.

The metaphysics underpinning Chinese medicine was subsequently highly developed by both the Daoist and Neo-Confucian schools during the Song dynasty, as exemplified in the Diagrams of the Supreme Ultimate (Figure 2.2) by Zhou Dunyi (1017–1023) and Chen Tuan (c.950). The uppermost circle in both diagrams represents the state of non-being, wú jí in Chinese (literally without a pole), which is the other face of Tài Jí (literally great pole). We can see that spirit (shén) is associated with the state of non-being (wú jí) in Chen's diagram in the upper right. There are many obvious references to the *Yi Jing* in these diagrams, but the dichotomy/identity between being and non-being had already been expressed in the *Dao De Jing* Chapter 40:

> "All things under heaven sprang from It (i.e., the Dao) as existing (and named); that existence sprang from It as non- existent (and not named)."[5]

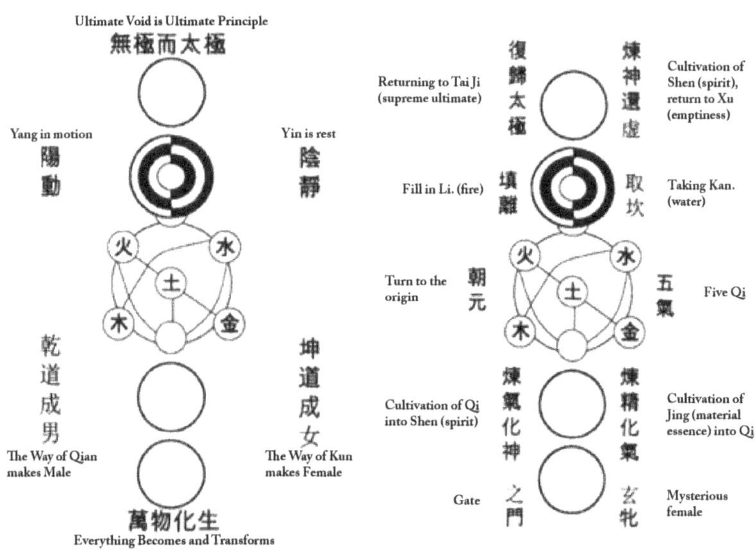

Figure 2.2 Taijitu and Wujitu, being and non-being
Source: Robin Wang

5 ctext.org/dao-de-jing 天下萬物生於有，有生於無.

From a practical point of view, the state of non-being, which is the abode of spirit, was recognized as the source of becoming and transformation (Zhou's lowest circle), processes that are ideally the target or goal of classical acupuncture treatment (stated more explicitly in the formal medical texts), but can be traced back to Lao Zi's classic.

Chapter 42 presents another interesting parallel between the *Dao De Jing* and the *Yi Jing*:

> "Tao produces unity; unity produces duality; duality produces trinity; trinity produces all things.
>
> All things bear the negative principle (yin) and embrace the positive principle (yang). Immaterial vitality, the third principle (chi), makes them harmonious."[6]

I believe we can read the later Neo-Confucian viewpoint as being pre-figured in these earlier texts as follows: the Dao exists at the level of non-being (wú jí). It produces undifferentiated (unitary) being (tài jí). Tài jí produces yin/yang, which in turn produces trinity, often represented as Heaven/Man/Earth, from which all creation becomes manifest by differentiation. It is possible to see in the above passage an analogy to the monograms, bigrams, and trigrams of the *Yi Jing*. In practice, the hexagrams of the *Yi Jing* are almost always interpreted in terms of their component trigrams, illustrating one step in this differentiation from trinity into totality.

6 Goddard's translation: www.yellowbridge.com/onlinelit/daodejing42.php. Legge's translation of the first sentence (The Dao produced One; One produced Two; Two produced Three; Three produced All things) is more familiar to English readers, but seems to me to miss the significance of the ordinal nature of numbers present in Goddard, and also lacks the implication that this is an ongoing, ever-present process, not something that happened in some ancient past. Tao is the Wade transliteration of Dao, and chi is the Wade transliteration of qi. 道生一, 一生二, 二生三, 三生萬物. 萬物負陰而抱陽, 沖氣以為和.

The intention of the founders of TCM, as mentioned in the introduction, of removing all matters relating to spirit, non-being, and metaphysics in general seems to me to be in direct conflict with the very essence of the type of classical thought from which acupuncture developed. Any attempt to establish the reality and importance of spirit and non-being by evidence-based research is likely to be doomed to failure, which is certainly one of the reasons for the tensions that developed in the West in the twentieth century between practitioners trained in Worsley's Five Element style of practice, with its emphasis on spirit, mind, and emotions, and the more materialist approach of TCM promulgated by the Chinese authorities.

Let us examine, by returning to the original text of *Lao Zi*, whether there might be, even in this early work, a hint that an Eastern scientific (i.e., inductive, qualitative, and synthetic) viewpoint was being espoused. One of the more poetic and also mystical chapters, number 21, reads (Blakney 1980, p.42):

> "The omnipresent Virtue will take shape
> According only to the Way.
> The Way itself is like something
> Seen in a dream, elusive, evading one,
> In it are things like shadows in twilight.
> In it are essences, subtle but real,
> Embedded in truth."[7]

If we take the Dao to be natural law, it is obvious that this axiomatic underpinning of reality is not something that would be directly visible, but only observable through its manifestations. Virtue (德 Dé) is acting as this intermediary. Where do we draw the line between things that can be directly observed, and those that must be inferred from our observations? Like dreams, we cannot observe

7 ctext.org/dao-de-jing 孔德之容, 唯道是從. 道之為物, 唯恍唯惚. 忽兮恍兮, 其中有象; 恍兮忽兮, 其中有物. 窈兮冥兮, 其中有精; 其精甚真, 其中有信.

those of others directly, and yet we all recognize their reality. One category of the fundamental substances composing the human organism are the Essences (精 Jīng), which are here stated to be subtle (perhaps not directly observable), but real nonetheless. I am impressed by Blakney's paraphrase of this chapter:

> "There is a virtue, a power that issues from the Way like a magnetic field around a magnet. As the magnet controls the shape of the field, so the Way controls its virtue or power." (Blakney 1980, p.42)

Blakney uses this analogy of magnetism again in paraphrasing chapter 25:

> "I do not know its name;
> A name for it is 'Way';
> Pressed for designation,
> I call it Great.
> Great means outgoing,
> Outgoing, far-reaching
> Far-reaching, return."[8]

> "The Way…is not a phenomenon, but the description… suggests the lines of force in a magnetic field. They go out from one pole and return to the other." (Blakney 1980, p.50)

One reason I am citing Blakney's use of magnetism to interpret *Lao Zi* is that the originator of Archaic Acupuncture, Dr. Igor Simonov, alludes to the magnetic impact of the sun on the earth to explain the observations enunciated by early Chinese acupuncture practitioners in the *Nan Jing*. This will be discussed in Chapter 6, but I point it out here to underscore the possibility

---

8 ctext.org/dao-de-jing 吾不知其名, 字之曰道, 強為之名曰大. 大曰逝, 逝曰遠, 遠曰反.

that the earliest strata of Chinese medicine were plausibly based on "scientific" observations and hypotheses.

A major difference between Western and Oriental sciences has been mentioned above: the former is materialist in its philosophy, while the latter insists that there is a deeper level of reality beyond the material one. *Lao Zi* 39 contains multiple examples of this non-materialist philosophy (Blakney 1980, p.78):

> "The sky (天 Heaven) obtained it (the Dao) and was clarified;
> The earth (地) received it and was settled firm;
> The spirits (神 Shén) got it and were energized (靈 Líng)…
> All things, as they partook it came alive (生 Shēng)."[9]

Interestingly, a concluding remark near the end of chapter 39 sounds as if it could have been written by a contemporary philosopher grappling with the nature of "science":

> "Truly, a cart is more than the sum of its parts." (Blakney 1980, p.78)[10]

Limiting "science" to materialism alone leaves it with considerable difficulty when confronted by the obvious existence of emergent properties, exemplified here in the cart, an object that cannot be explained by simply deconstructing it into its parts. The central problem with the limits of Western science mentioned earlier, how to explain mind and consciousness, also has to do with this same issue of emergent properties.

9 ctext.org/dao-de-jing 天得一以清; 地得一以寧; 神得一以靈; 谷得一以盈; 萬物得一以生.

10 故至數輿無輿. (Following Ma Wang Dui B.)

Chapter 3

Huái Nán Zǐ 淮南子

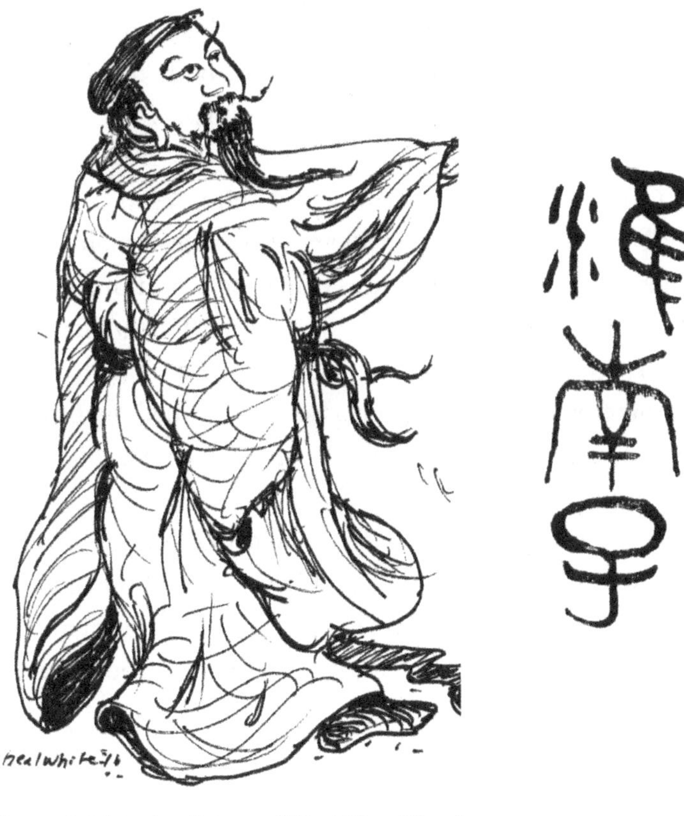

Figure 3.1 Liu An, Prince of Huai Nan. The characters on the right are the Seal script writing of Huai Nan Zi

Source: Neal White and Peter Eckman

In order to understand the way in which Oriental medical theory can be seen as using an inductive, qualitative, and synthetic (as opposed to deductive, quantitative, and analytic) approach to the scientific investigation of natural law, one has to deal with its axiomatic premises. To my mind, its most important axiom, the principle of resonance, was clearly stated in *Huai Nan Zi*. This text was a collaborative work written by scholars in the court of Liu An, the Prince of Huai Nan (Figure 3.1), some time before 139 BCE, making it roughly contemporaneous with the *Nei Jing*. These scholars were affiliated with the Huang Lao school of Daoism, a shamanic grouping from the State of Chŭ (楚).[1] The text consists of 21 chapters, from which I will focus on chapter 6, where the concept of resonance is both clearly stated, and illustrated via a number of specific examples.

Before presenting the thesis put forth in *Huai Nan Zi* chapter 6, I would like to explain why I think resonance is the most basic axiom of Oriental medicine. There are certainly other candidates that one could choose as being the most fundamental, including Yin/Yang, Five Elements, Heaven/Earth/Man, and Qì. The first three of these are actually corollaries based on this principle of resonance, while Qì is best seen as the medium through which resonance operates. Resonance can also be seen to account for the action of both acupuncture and herbs, as well as other modalities of Oriental medicine. To give just one example, each of the classical acupuncture points has at least one traditional name, whose meaning can be used in selecting points for treatment. This approach has been called the "Spirit of the Point," and is widely

1 As in the *Chŭ Cí—Songs of Chŭ* (楚辭). Many of these songs or poems depict the mystical flight of the Shaman to the Source, the Dao.

used in many styles of acupuncture.[2] This method presumably works because of the resonance between the nature of what is lacking in the pathological state of the patient, as expressed in the totality of signs and symptoms, and the corresponding normal physiological state that the practitioner wishes to evoke in the patient, in order to encourage a return to healthy functioning. There is a very interesting connection in this regard between the concepts of Spirit and of resonance, both of which exist at the level of wú jí (i.e., non-material).

Huai Nan Zi was not the earliest Chinese work to mention resonance, but rather the *locus classicus* for its detailed explanation. The *Yi Jing* refers to resonance in its commentary on the first Hexagram (Qian) attributed to Confucius:

> "The Master said: Notes of the same key 'respond' to one another; creatures of the same nature seek one another; water flows towards the place that is (low and) damp; fire rises up towards what is dry; clouds follow the dragon, and winds follow the tiger: (so) the sage makes his appearance, and all men look to him. Things that draw their origin from heaven move towards what is above; things that draw their origin

2 One of the most thorough presentations of the "Spirit of the Points" can be found in Ellis, Wiseman, and Boss (1989), *Grasping the Wind.* This text is written by authors identified with the pre-TCM branch of acupuncture transmitted by James Tin Yau So, and I'm sure it subliminally influenced my choice of title for the present treatise. It is, however, based entirely on classical Chinese references, including the Preface quotation of Sun Si Miao, "The names of the points are not merely nominal; each has a profound meaning." O'Connor and Bensky (1981), a more definitive TCM work, makes passing reference to the significance of point names on p.139. See also Worsley (1982, pp.110–112), Connelly (1979, p.168), Lavier (1966, pp.245–248), and Kespi (2012).

> from the earth cleave to what is below—so does everything follow its kind."[3]

In this passage, "respond" is a translation of the Chinese characters xiāng yìng 相應, forming one of several terms (compound or singular) that are all more or less synonymous, and which I render as either "correspond" or "resonance" depending on the grammatical context. The other common synonyms are xiāng gǎn 相感 and gǎn yìng 感應, the last of which has become the standard, following *Huai Nan Zi*. Even the singular character gǎn 感 can carry the meaning of correspond/resonance, as in this quote from Needham:

> A 5th century author Shih Shuo Hsin Yu wrote, "Mr. Yin, a native of Chinchao once asked a (Taoist) monk Chan Yeh-Yuan, what is the fundamental idea of the *I Ching*? The latter answered, the fundamental idea of the *I Ching* can be expressed in one word, Gan (Resonance)." (Needham 1956, p.304)

The title of *Huai Nan Zi* chapter 6 is "Lǎn Míng Xùn" 覽冥訓, which has been translated as "Peering into the Obscure" (Le Blanc 1985, p.102),[4] but which I think might be better rendered as "Lecture on Perceiving the Unseen World." Does either of these translations sound like it could be a "scientific" treatise? Let us examine the classical characters to see if my translation is justified:

---

3 http://ctext.org/book-of-changes/gan1. This is Legge's translation of 同聲相應,同氣相求.水流濕,火就燥,雲從龍,風從虎,聖人作而萬物覩.本乎天者親上,本乎地者親下,則各從其類也.

4 My discussion of *Huai Nan Zi* chapter 6 is essentially based on Le Blanc's pioneering work. Le Blanc was a student of the late Claude Larre, who was also my first teacher of how to learn to read Chinese characters.

Lăn 覽: to look at, inspect, perceive or distinguish. It is used in the expression, "to understand it all in one glance" (Mathews 1979, 3804).

Míng 冥: dark, obscure, the unseen world, deep, profound (Mathews 1979, 4528).

Xùn 訓: to instruct, to lecture, to admonish, to counsel (Mathews 1979, 2914).

Putting these characters together, we may have a sense that "in one glance" we understand the nature of the unseen (wu ji) world, via an inductive mode of cognition. We see the effects, we infer the mechanisms. This could be the title of a treatise on magnetism or gravity, although from a qualitative rather than a quantitative perspective. These are phenomena we accept in Western science, even though we don't always know how they act. Chapter 6 gives us reasoned advice on how to understand the axiomatic operative mechanism that exists at the non-material level of nature, which it identifies as resonance (găn yìng):

> "The mutual response (gan ying) of things belonging in the same category (lei) is darkly mysterious (xuan miao) and extremely subtle (shen wei). Knowledge (zhi) cannot explain it, nor discussion (bian) unravel it. Each thing is affected (gan) inasmuch as it resembles or partakes of the shapes and categories (xing lei) of other things."

This translation by Le Blanc uses two English words (mutual response) for two Chinese characters (găn yìng), instead of the more concise term (resonance) with which it is synonymous, and which Le Blanc adopts later in his translation of Chapter 6 (Le Blanc 1985, p.192). This short excerpt is loaded with significance for anyone interested in understanding the Eastern, as opposed to the Western, mode of scientific discussion.

Therefore I will examine the key terms, which were indicated by pinyin transcriptions in the quotation.

Gǎn 感 means "moved to response through the feelings and affections; induction" (Mathews 1979, 3232). The reference to feelings and affections supports the association of resonance and Spirit as related terms (further suggested by the use of the Heart radical in gǎn). On the other hand, the reference to "induction" allows for an Eastern scientific viewpoint, as emphatically put forward in the writings of Manfred Porkert, one of the first Western scholars to characterize Chinese medicine as a science, based on inductive synthesis (Porkert 1995).[5] In addition to the Heart radical, the character for gǎn includes parts that mean battle axe, mouth, and wound. The mouth wounds by biting, like a halberd biting into flesh. So there is some action (biting) associated with emotions (Heart). The combined picture is of something being induced to move by a subtle influence (Heart/emotion). My interpretation of this character implies that resonance works by some mechanism that cannot be materially explained, like the shén 神 of the Heart. The most common usages of gǎn are in phrases where it means "to contract" or "be affected by." For example, there is a medical use of gǎn in the expression gǎn mào 感冒 for catching a cold or flu. Here, being bitten makes sense, reminiscent of the teeth pictured in the character xié 邪 of xié qì 邪氣.[6] The *Nei Jing* uses the terms gǎn xié and xiāng gǎn 相感,[7]

5 See also Porkert's detailed thesis at www.jungtao.edu/index.php/classical-chinese-medicine/resources?id=44.

6 Xié qì is the Chinese term for pathogenic factors.

7 *Su Wen* 81: "Water and Fire xiāng gǎn (水火相感)." *Ling Shu* 5: "Heaven and Earth xiāng gǎn (天地相感)." There is a slight difference in connotation between gǎn yīng and xiāng gǎn, as shown in these citations. Xiāng gǎn means mutually affect, which could include "oppose each other," while gǎn yīng would have the more strict meaning of resonate.

but not gǎn yīng 感應, which didn't become the standard expression for resonance until later.

Yìng 應 by itself means "must, necessary, proper, fitting, right, suitable, reply, respond, echo, correspond, fulfill, be fulfilled." It also carries other connotations suggested by its use in phrases such as "should at once, it is my duty immediately, respond without the slightest hesitation, to answer a call, to obey the will of Heaven and be in harmony with men, the clocks struck at the proper time (i.e., tuned, synchronized), the tides came at the proper time without fail, to be in correspondence with all things" (Mathews 1979, 7477). Compared to gǎn, yìng is found much more often in the *Nei Jing*, where it typically means "correspond." For example, yìng is used there to indicate that a certain pulse pattern corresponds to a particular stage of illness.[8]

Additional passages where yìng refers to correspondence include, "The arrangements of Heaven and Earth are what humans' Shén-Spirit corresponds to,"[9] and "Heaven is Yang, the Earth is Yin, the sun is Yang, the moon is Yin. Longer months and shorter months, 360 days make up one year. Humans correspond to this too."[10] Note the use of yìng as the operator in these passages referring to correspondence. Another example of this usage of yìng can be found in herbal medicine in the expression "ying yen liang fang," which means a good prescription, that is, one that corresponds to the symptom complex. Often yìng is part of the compound term xiāng yìng 相應 (mutually correspond), as in *Nan Jing* Difficulty 13, which

---

8 *Su Wen* 20: "When the pulses above and below, left and right correspond (相應) to each other…the disease is severe. When above and below, left and right do not conform…death." 上下左右之脈相應如參舂者, 病甚上下左右相失不可數者, 死.

9 *Su Wen* 74: 天地之大紀, 人神之通應也.

10 *Su Wen* 6: 天為陽, 地為陰, 日為陽, 月為陰, 大小月三百六十日成一歲, 人亦應之.

states, "complexion and pulse must mutually correspond."[11] Difficulty 13 goes on to elaborate: "The five viscera have their respective corresponding (yìng 應) voice, facial color, smell, and flavor, which should correspond to the pulse at the wrist and the skin along the ulna as well. If not, it means presence of disease." This passage is very close to the "color, sound, odor, and emotion" (CSOE) methodology taught in Worsley's Five Element style of acupuncture based on constitutional diagnosis, except that Worsley substituted emotion for flavor. Worsley's choice here is understandable: all of the other correspondences are signs that can be detected by examination, while flavor preference cannot. The emotion that belongs in this set of Elemental correspondences is an observable sign, and is stated many times in the classics. If we ponder the importance of this character "yìng 應" in Five Element teachings, some interesting associations can be found. Yìng is composed of two parts: a radical and a phonetic. The Heart (心) is the radical, which connects with the idea of feelings, Spirit and the realm of wú jí. The phonetic is (yīng) the falcon, a tame bird that serves man, and that originally had a connotation of suddenness (Wieger 1965, p.335, lessons 168 J and K). The complete meaning of yìng 應 is thus to immediately correspond or resonate.

11 "Complexion and (movement in the) vessels must be compared as to their mutual correspondence (相應)" (Unschuld 1986, p.170).

What do birds (as in the phonetic component of yìng) have to do with acupuncture? Is it a coincidence that one of the legendary founders of Chinese medicine, Bian Que 扁鵲 (Flat Magpie) (Buck 2015, pp.72–74),[12] famous for his skill in applying acupuncture, was depicted in Han dynasty stone carvings as half man and half bird, as in Figure 3.2? If the goal of acupuncture treatment is to foster a resonance between the point treated and the normal physiology that needs to be restored, then the sudden cures attributed to Bian Que can be understood as analogous to the suddenness of the falcon. As a personal observation, I have often been amazed at the seemingly instant response to accurate acupuncture treatment, both in its effects on the symptoms and its effects on the pulse, returning the latter from a pathological to a normal state.

The common thread that ties together all the various usages of yìng is its meaning conveyed by the terms correspondence or resonance, which were understood as occurring via a non-material mechanism.

12 Bian Que's traditional dating is 407–310 BCE. He is credited with introducing the four examinations of Chinese medicine: looking, listening–smelling, questioning, and palpating. Buck presents an interesting hypothesis, that Bian Que was a collective name for members of a medical clan that used these diagnostic methods and their associated medical lore to distinguish themselves from shamanic healers. This idea would explain how Bian Que could be referred to by Sima Qian in 75 BCE as living during the dates mentioned, but was also later credited with authorship of the *Nan Jing*, which wasn't written until the first century CE.

(a)

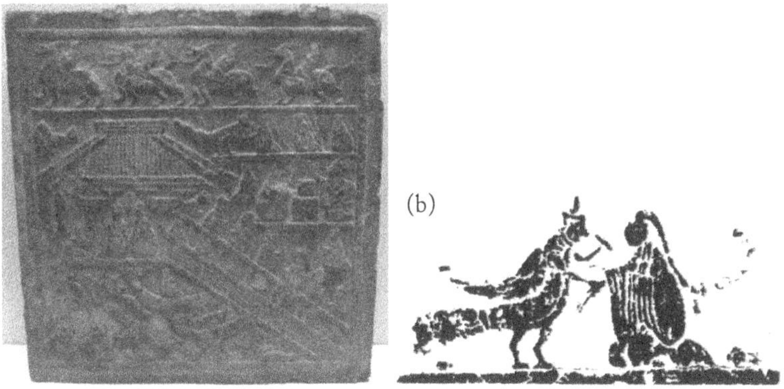

(b)

Figure 3.2 Bian Que[13] (a) Stone carving from the Eastern Han Dynasty; (b) detailed view
Source: commons.wikimedia.org

Having established the importance of gǎn yìng (resonance) as an axiom of Chinese medicine, let us return to the *Huai Nan Zi* quotation, in order to understand what the Han dynasty authors had to say about it. In my mind there is a parallel between the use of two characters (gǎn and yìng) to convey the concept of resonance, and the two aspects that resonance implies.

The first aspect is indicated by the term lèi 類 (Mathews 1979, 4244), which means a category, class, or kind, and is used in reasoning by analogy—things that are similar or alike. It appears in the title of the *Classic of Categories* (*Lei Jing*) by Zhang Jie Bin (1624), an attempt to organize the *Nei Jing*'s content in a more "reader friendly" fashion. Categories are stated in *Huai Nan Zi* as being the objects of resonance. We can see the application of this idea in all the basic theories of Chinese medicine, as exemplified by Yin/Yang or by Five Phases.

13 Stone carving unearthed at Liangcheng, Weishan, Shandong Province. Towards the upper right corner one can see the divine healer Bian Que 扁鵲 (depicted as a bird with a human head) treating three sick people, using acupuncture.

Both of these theories depend on first establishing lists of members that resonate with one of their categories. For example, Yin includes all things dark, cold, inside, feminine, and so on, while Yang includes all things bright, hot, outside, and masculine. The Fire phase includes all things bitter, red, scorched, and joyful, while the Metal phase includes all things pungent, white, rotten, and sad. It is from these categories that we can understand the Heart as the Yin (interior) Organ system of the Fire (hot, red) phase and the Lung as the Yin (interior) Organ system of the Metal (white, sad—as in the classical description of tuberculosis patients) phase. The lists given can be expanded infinitely, membership being governed simply by resonant associations.

The second aspect of resonance is not the assignment to categories, but rather the actions or effects that all members of a category resonantly display. For example, all things Yin have oppositional effects to all things Yang, but at the same time they also gradually transform into Yang. Thus night becomes day and winter becomes summer, even though they have opposite qualities. The Fire phase gives birth to the Earth phase, while simultaneously restraining the Metal phase. There are many texts that expand these illustrative examples voluminously, for those who are interested.

Huai Nan Zi goes on to state that the phenomenon of resonance is darkly mysterious (xuán miào) and extremely subtle (shēn wēi). Knowledge (zhī) cannot explain it, nor discussion (biàn) unravel it. My understanding of these two sentences is that the authors are claiming axiomatic status for gǎn yìng, meaning that it is a truth about nature that can be inferred from observations, but cannot be further analyzed. The Chinese characters point to this interpretation of the intention of the Han dynasty authors. Xuán 玄 (Mathews 1979, 2881) meaning dark, depicts a thread dyed black. This character is frequently used in Daoist writings to refer to the ineffable. Miào 妙 (Mathews 1979, 4474) meaning wonderful (full of wonder), when combined with xuán (which is also its radical), means subtle and mysterious. Shēn 深, translated here as extremely, also connotes deep, abstruse, and profound. It has the character for water as its radical, which carries similar connotations in English, as in "the watery depths." For the Han Chinese, Water was not only deep and mysterious, but also black in terms of resonant color, echoing xuán. Wēi 微 (Mathews 1979, 7061) means subtle, but also minute, obscure, and hidden. It is used in modern Chinese to refer to microbes, corpuscles, and capillaries, that is, objects too small to actually see. In the classical medical texts, subtle often refers to the Essences (Jīng), which are at the origin of creation, and the material partner of the Spirit (Shén). We can see that these four characters have interlocking connections with each other, which is both poetic and at the same time a specific example of resonance at play.

The next sentence (Knowledge (zhī) cannot explain it, nor discussion (biàn) unravel it) establishes the axiomatic status of gǎn yìng. Zhī 知 (Mathews 1979, 932) means to know, to perceive. The character depicts an arrow fixed in its target. Wieger explains this as "knowledge makes a man able to give an opinion, rapid and precise as an arrow hitting its mark" (Wieger 1965, p.300, lesson 131 E). Biàn 辯 (Mathews 1979, 5242) means to discuss, argue, explain. It is an interesting character depicting two criminals impeaching each other. To me, this character conveys the understanding that explanations are always tentative conclusions, and should be considered as hypotheses, rather than as ultimate truths. So *Huai Nan Zi*'s conclusion is that this mysterious phenomenon of resonance cannot be known by any kind of rational analysis based on evidence presented in a discussion. Rather, it is an immanent aspect of nature that is subject to neither proof nor disproof.

The final sentence in this excerpt from chapter 6, "Each thing is affected (gǎn) inasmuch as it resembles or partakes of the shapes and categories (xíng lèi) of other things," introduces one new character, xíng 形 (Mathews 1979, 2759). This character, meaning form or shape, has the same pronunciation as the character for Phases or Elements in the Five Element theory, and so is ideal for describing the resonance between members of the same Element set. In the West we call this observation (significance of shape) the Doctrine of Signatures. Some, like Needham and Unschuld, may consider the Doctrine of Signatures magical thinking, but it is very similar to modern scientific notions of fractals and holograms.

Let me summarize what has been presented so far regarding the meaning of gǎn yìng by citing the translations of other authors. Mathews defines gǎn yìng as moved to response through the feelings, or induction. Le Blanc translates gǎn yìng as either resonance, or stimulus and response. Bodde translates gǎn yìng as action and reaction.[14] All three of these translations seem compatible with a scientific perspective: induction, stimulus and response, and action and reaction. However, *Huai Nan Zi* warns us that attempting to understand the mechanism of gǎn yìng is fruitless (knowledge cannot explain it), but that doesn't mean we shouldn't ponder the mystery, remembering that the Heart radical is in both terms. Are the multiple appearances of the Heart radical a hint that there is a connection to Mind and Spirit? There are two sayings in Chinese that discuss the

14 Le Blanc (1985), p.xii of the Foreword, written by Derk Bodde, Professor Emeritus of Chinese Studies, University of Pennsylvania. Bodde was a thesis advisor for Le Blanc.

relationship of form (xíng 形) and Spirit (Shén 神): "The body is the material form of the Spirit," and "having the form, but lacking the Spirit" (Mathews 1979, p.413). These terms are not coequal, but are manifestations of a hierarchical relationship. Chapter 1 of *Huai Nan Zi* states:

> "Thus, when the spirit rules, the body follows and benefits from this. When the body governs, the spirit follows and is harmed by this." (Major *et al.* 2010, p.76)

Is it too bizarre to suppose that all of creation has some kind of non-material life? If indeed homeopathy also works by resonance, isn't it interesting that the mental and emotional pictures of the remedies, even the mineral ones, are considered to be more crucial than the physical ones in differential diagnosis?

The pre-*Nei Jing* Chinese literature clearly recognized the phenomenon of resonance, as seen in multiple passages about vibrating lute strings, but other acoustical phenomena demonstrating resonance were also recognized, as in *Guan Zi* (3rd century BCE): "In antiquity, Huang Di generated the 5 tones on the basis of the slow and fast (soundings), thereby ordering the 5 bells. Once he had regulated the 5 tones, he established the 5 Agents to order the Heavenly seasons, and then he set up the 5 official ranks to order the positions of Man" (Unschuld and Tessenow 2011, p.103; see Figure 3.3).

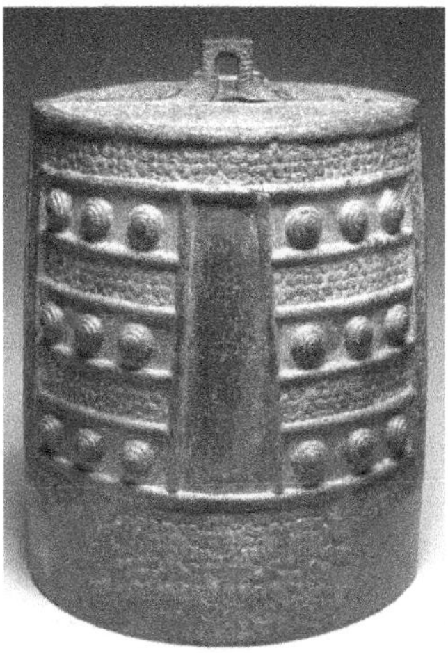

Figure 3.3 Chinese bells[15]
Source: Walters Art Museum

References to the resonance of lute strings appear in the following texts. In the *Yi Jing*, "Notes of the same kind respond to one another." *Zhuang Zi*, "The Yang sound Kung evokes its correspondent. And so for the Yin sound (Chiao)" (Watson 1964, 24/158, pp.267–268). The *Chunqiu Fan Lu* also includes a reference to the resonating of lutes. However, it is in the *Huai Nan Zi* that we find the most detailed description of this phenomenon: "When the lute tuner strikes the Kung note (on one instrument), the Kung note (on the other) responds. When he plucks the Chiao note (on one), the Chiao note (on the other) vibrates. Now (let us assume that) someone changes the tuning

15 The emperor Huizong (reigned 1100–1126) was anxious to bring ritual court music into accordance with ancient standards. Taking the length of the emperor's fingers as a guide, the fundamental pitch was determined (it turned out to be almost exactly middle C). New sets of bells were then cast, their form based on a newly excavated set dating from about the 5th century BC. On each bell, the name of the pitch was engraved on one side and characters meaning "Bureau of Music" on the other. Image: https://upload.wikimedia.org/wikipedia/commons/e/ec/Chinese_-_Bell_-_Walters_542185.jpg.

of one string in such a way that it does not match any of the 5 notes, and by striking it, sets all 25 strings resonating. In this case, there has as yet been no differentiation as regards sound... That sound which governs all musical notes has been evoked" (Le Blanc 1985, p.138).

Clearly, this passage takes the concept of resonance and develops it further. In fact, Le Blanc uses the terms "relative resonance" and "total resonance" to differentiate these two phenomena. For me, total resonance evokes the idea of the proper situation of the Heart as being empty. *When the Heart is empty it can respond (resonate) to any input, but if it is already pre-occupied its ability to respond is restricted.* A quote from Needham supports this interpretation: "Scholars of old-time said that the mind is originally empty, and only because of this can it respond to natural things (yìng wù) without prejudices. Only the empty mind can respond to the things of nature. Though everything resonates with the mind, the mind should be as if it had never resonated, and things should not remain on it" (Needham 1956, p.89). It is important to note that the same Chinese character 心 xīn means both Heart and mind.

In summary, there are two kinds of resonance, both described in *Huai Nan Zi* as manifestations of gǎn yìng. The "exoteric" meaning of gǎn yìng is "like influences like," what Le Blanc calls "relative resonance." His explanation is that "All things in the universe are interrelated and influence each other according to pre-set patterns, so that interaction appears as spontaneous and not caused by an external agent." On the other hand, the "esoteric" meaning of gǎn yìng is that "everything is one," which Le Blanc calls "total resonance." He paraphrases *Huai Nan Zi* thus: "All things relate, not because they share the same category, but because the universe, on the deepest level, is fundamentally one—the Supreme Ultimate (Tài Jí)."

Let me illustrate these different types of resonance, using the actual examples presented in *Huai Nan Zi* (Le Blanc 1985, p.8). "The Sun mirror which produces (gathers) Fire (both share the Yang category) and the moon mirror which collects Water (both share the Yin category) display relative resonance" ("like influences like"). The converse ("unlike does not influence unlike") is also an aspect of relative resonance. The example given is, "while a lodestone (natural magnet) attracts iron, it does not attract tile (ceramic, clay)." Relative resonance is an easy concept to understand, regardless of whether or not one believes it is a law of nature. Total resonance, on the other hand, is not as easy to grasp. *Huai Nan Zi* uses the categories it already described in discussing relative resonance (Fire and Water) to illustrate total resonance thus: "And yet, if it were within the (power) to gather (things within) one category from Tài Jí, then one could immediately produce Fire and Water." Since both have a common origin (in Tài Jí), Fire and Water, though ostensibly different, share another kind of resonance that expresses an even deeper law of nature, but one that perhaps is only apparent to mystics. Who has this ability to tune a lute string so that striking it will vibrate all 25 strings? By what "power" can one gather opposing members of a category, like Fire and Water, and produce both from the same source?

Le Blanc attempts to address these questions. He starts with a classical epigram, "Yin and Yang share a common Qì, and move each other." From this he continues, "Things that belong to the same category and share a common substance have the power to influence one another, respond to one another, and resound together (gǎn yìng) precisely because Qì serves as a medium or continuum through which movement and change, following the alternation of Yin and Yang, can be actualized." Finally, he adds, "Only one kind of Qì however has universal extension and unlimited efficacy—the Qì of Dào... This Qì is that which

Huai Nan Zi refers to as subtle essence, subtle energy and spiritual essence. At the level of the most subtle essence, gǎn yìng operates as a universal pattern, linking and transcending even Yin and Yang. This is the mystical total resonance of being at one with the Dào" (Le Blanc 1985, pp.129 and 204). In other words, total resonance "is based on the persistent affinity and attraction of things that were originally one, but that became scattered when the world began. Through the True Man, gǎn yìng recreates the original unity." This is an organismic view of the universe. Originally it was whole, but when it became separated it retained these ties due to resonating categories. We are left with more than one mystery, however: how do the two aspects of gǎn yìng relate to each other, and what did the authors of *Huai Nan Zi* mean by "the True Man"?

Starting with the first question, is there some way of understanding these two different aspects of gǎn yìng that would allow us to see resonance as a fundamental axiom of nature that includes both? Here is Le Blanc's viewpoint: "We may define gǎn yìng as the power of things to affect and be affected in such a way as to bring about harmony" (Le Blanc 1985, p.209). This is perhaps best exemplified by the anecdotal lute strings. Sympathetic vibration and harmony (harmonics) are seen as the basis of energy or vibrational medicine. Illness is seen as being out of tune, or as a loss of harmony. Medicines (herbs/needles), from this point of view, act to tune our instruments (organisms) by supplying the authentic vibration, and we resonate to that with a reawakening of original nature endowed to us at conception, but originating in Tài Jí. Acoustic vibrations are of course the essence of music. Perhaps not surprisingly, the ancient characters for medicine and music are much the same, leading to the saying, "Medicine is music, music is medicine," as illustrated in Figure 3.4.

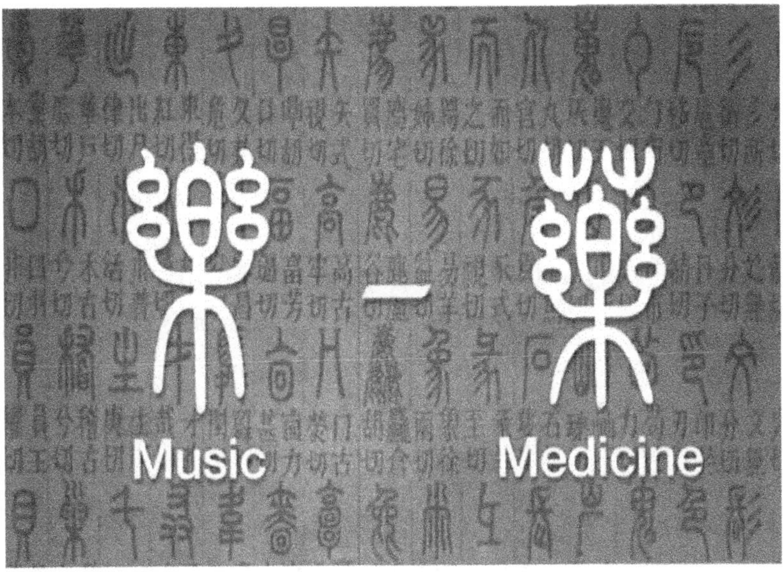

Figure 3.4 Ancient characters for music and medicine[16]
Source: ShenYunPerformingArts.org

Next we come to the question of who is "the True Man"? In this regard I find it amusing that Western scholars seem comfortable with the term "political science" and yet object to the notion of "Oriental medical science." In the West we like to draw sharp boundaries between disciplines, such as science, religion, and politics, whereas in the East there is a more fluid continuum between them. Le Blanc is astute in recognizing that the discussion of total resonance supplies the justification for all the preceding attention to relative resonance. He points out that the authors were not merely speculative philosophers, but were court retainers

16 The character on the left was the Seal script for 樂 yuè (yao in Wade-Giles), meaning music. According to Wieger (1965, p.224), it represents a 木 wooden support on which a 白 drum and 幺 bells are hung. The same character, when pronounced lè (lao in Wade-Giles), means the effect produced by music, i.e., pleasure or joy. The Seal script character on the right 藥 yào simply adds the plant radical 艸 implying an early recognition that medicines act in the same manner as music, i.e., via resonance.

to the Prince of Huai Nan, and were expected to come up with something practical to justify their keep. What they concluded was, "The most perfect government is that of non-action (wú wéi), for it operates through the natural (zì rán) resonance (gǎn yìng) of all things. The perfect ruler is the True Man (zhēn rén) who, being one with the Dao is in a state of mutual resonance with all things" (Le Blanc 1985, p.192). Thus it is the King (perfect ruler) who has this mysterious "power" of total resonance, and by including this "political science" explanation of the meaning of kingship, justifies the whole compilation of *Huai Nan Zi* as a gift of great worth from the Prince to the King.

It is doubtful whether anyone in the 21st century still believes in the "divine right of kings," which is more or less the Western complement to *Huai Nan Zi*'s "True Man." Does that situation invalidate the idea of total resonance as a law of nature? Not necessarily. I have already cited the interpretation of total resonance as being the potential of an "empty Heart/Mind (xīn)." There is no need to be a king or emperor in order to achieve this state, but perhaps it is an equally difficult accomplishment, for who among us can approach each moment without any preconceptions or prejudices? Most religions and other spiritual traditions share this goal, either implicitly or explicitly. Meditation is one technique shared by these various spiritual traditions aimed at achieving this state.

I have often wondered about the absence of any discussion of love in the Chinese medical classics, given their extensive references to the other human emotions in health and illness. Of course, the word "love" can be used to describe many different experiences, but I think a case can be made for the equivalence of the Chinese empty Heart's ability to be in total resonance with all of creation and at least some of the Western religions' teachings about God's love for all of creation. Despite the fact that the medical classics did not discuss love, other roughly contemporaneous Chinese philosophers did. For instance, Mo Zi (c.400 BCE) was a proponent of the idea of "Universal Love" (博愛 bó ài), which sounds to me like a parallel concept to the Western spiritual beliefs. Moreover, later Chinese medical theorists began to explicitly discuss the importance of love, or lack thereof, as an etiological factor to be considered in diagnosis. Sun Si Miao wrote that people suffer illness "because they do not have love in their life, and are not cherished."[17] In this case Sun's connotation of love would be much closer to what we mean by the word in a Western secular context. I'm not sure, however, that we need to insist on an absolute distinction between these two connotations of love, especially in the practice of medicine. Since love is not included in the classical Seven Emotions, where does it fit in medical practice? I believe it is the essence of the ideal practitioner–patient relationship, in which the practitioner's Heart is able to totally resonate with everything the patient presents, because his/her Heart is empty of preconceptions. It is not unreasonable to propose that the Chinese of classical times understood the relationship of the Heart to love, in much the same way as they understood total resonance. The character for love, ài 愛 (Mathews 1979, 9), has the Heart in its center. Wieger (1965) in Phonetic Series 721 lists the following characters as all pronounced the same (ài in the 4th tone): 僾 like/similar (reminiscent of lei-category), 曖 dull/obscure (reminiscent of xuan-obscure), 靉 cloudy/obscure (reminiscent of xuan-obscure), and 薆 to conceal (reminiscent of wei-hidden). It is highly unlikely to be coincidental that all these different characters derived from ài-love, and pronounced identically are found to parallel characters that are highlighted in *Huai Nan Zi* chapter 6.

17 Qian Jin Yi Fang, 682 CE, cited in Kaptchuk (2000, p.159).

In concluding my remarks regarding *Huai Nan Zi* chapter 6, I have some speculations about how the issues I've presented find expression in the clinical practice of Chinese medicine. Mostly we work with relative resonance—which point, which herb? To determine this we need to know the resonant categories. The dosage (strength and number of acupuncture points stimulated, or the quantity of herbs) depends on the sensitivity of the resonating instrument (i.e., the patient's unique nature). However, the love we treat our patients with is an example of using total resonance, which we are all capable of doing to a greater or lesser degree. It is my impression that with acupuncture at least, we don't always need to be technically perfect (relative resonance-wise) for treatment to be beneficial. Treatments given from a heart of love may work via a different means than those based on relative resonance. It is not beyond my imagination to suppose that a heightened access to total resonance could explain the miraculous healing powers of saints, sages, and other holy folk.

Chapter 4

Sù Wèn 素問

SIMPLE QUESTIONS

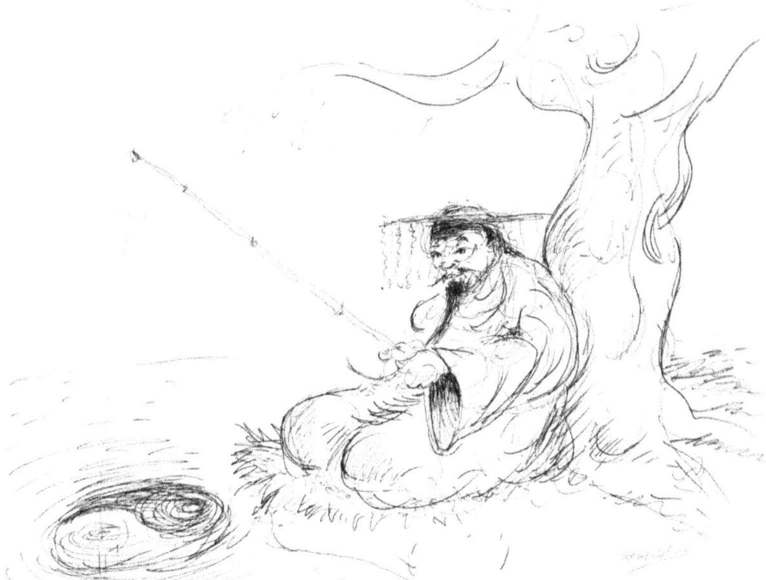

Figure 4.1 Huang Di (The Yellow Emperor)[1]
Source: Neal White

1 The legendary Yellow Emperor was considered the honorary author of the "Bible" of Chinese medicine, *Huángdì Nèijīng* 黄帝内經, which text comprises mainly dialogs with the equally legendary doctor Qí Bó. The first half of this text, *Sù Wèn*, deals primarily with the philosophical basis of Chinese medicine, symbolized here by the tài jí tú, emblem of yīn and yáng.

The *Su Wen* is a text comprising the first half of *The Yellow Emperor's Inner Classic* (*Huángdì Nèijīng* 黄帝内經, a work of collective authorship putatively dated to the late second or early first century BCE), which is regarded as the "Bible of Chinese Medicine." The character sù 素 depicts raw silk, with implications of being plain, unadorned and of the essence, in other words relating to the original constitution of things (Mathews 1979, 5490). The silk pictograph it uses is also found in the character jīng 經 for classic, so there is a natural resonance between these two terms. Generally speaking then, the *Su Wen* presents the fundamental (unadorned, essential, and constitutive) teachings, both abstract and concrete, which lay the groundwork for the practice of acupuncture, a subject that receives more developed attention in the second half of this Bible, the *Ling Shu*, which I will discuss in Chapter 5. As in the previous chapters, I will pick one specific topic to examine here, but it is one that I believe has escaped the attention of many translators and commentators on this voluminous text.

As this is the first chapter to specifically discuss a Chinese medical text, I will start with a very practical question: What is the most unique, and yet universal, methodology characteristic of almost all the versions of acupuncture and the other therapeutic modalities that characterize Chinese medicine? I believe most practitioners would identify pulse diagnosis as fulfilling that role. Where did the knowledge of pulse diagnosis come from? Unfortunately, the origins of pulse diagnosis are lost in the mists (and myths) of prehistoric time. Even before the *Su Wen*, there were written accounts of interpreting pulse findings, such as that mentioned by Sima Qian in the biography of Chunyu Yi (c.216–150 BCE).[2] One problem with evaluating early Chinese

2 *Shi Ji* or *Records of the Historian* was written c.94 BCE. See Buck (2015, pp.98–102) for a synopsis of the career of Chunyu Yi. Buck relates that among the

medical texts in this regard is that the same character, mài 脈, can mean both pulse and the concept rendered in English as meridian, channel, or vessel. An example is in the Ma Wang Dui silk scroll called the *Maishu*, believed to antedate the *Su Wen*, which refers to 11 mài. The following quote nicely illustrates this double meaning:

> "Well over half of the symptoms associated with the eleven mài described in the Mawangdui channel texts, for example, are of pain or discomfort along the mài in question. After each of the eleven descriptions of the mài in *Maishu* there is a list of symptoms that is introduced with the phrase shì dòng zé bìng 是動則病 'when it moves/becomes agitated then there will be illness.' What 'moves/becomes agitated' is the pulse."[3]

The *Su Wen* hints at the ancient origin of pulse diagnosis when it mentions the Yellow Emperor's main teacher, Qi Bo, as citing the equally legendary figure Jiu Daiji (reputed to be a contemporary of Shen Nong) as establishing the standards for the complexions and pulses (which should resonate with each other in a state of health).[4] How can a pulse resonate with a complexion? Unfortunately, this passage in the *Su Wen* does not state the standards to be used in pulse examination, so we are left to speculate on the authors' meaning. Contemporary pulse diagnosis in Chinese medicine is routinely carried out by examining the radial artery pulses in the

---

texts that Chunyu Yi cited as being received from his teacher Cheng Yangqing was *Huangdi Bianque Mai Shu*, a pulse diagnosis text in two parts, one linked to Bian Que and the other to the Yellow Emperor. It is noteworthy that Chunyu Yi lived in the same Shandong province as the Bian Que clan, so that a lineage connection between the two would not be difficult to imagine. Chunyu Yi was quoted by Sima Qian as saying the following about his method of diagnosing and treating patients: "I always palpate their mai first, and then treat them."

3 www.ucl.ac.uk/histmed/downloads/ma_teaching/lo/c123_2.pdf.

4 *Su Wen* 13. See also Unschuld and Tessenow (2011, p.223, footnote 9).

region of the left and right wrists, although there are alternative methods employed by various non-mainstream, yet adamantly traditional, practitioners.[5] In fact, the *Su Wen* describes one of these alternative methods (comparing the carotid and radial arterial pulses) in more specific detail than it describes radial pulse diagnosis, leading to some controversy as to whether or not radial pulse diagnosis was routinely practiced by the Chinese physicians who compiled the *Su Wen*.[6] I believe that there is abundant evidence in the *Su Wen* to confirm that knowledge of radial pulse diagnosis was assumed, rather than being explicitly described by its authors, although they didn't present clear standards for its practice, for reasons that were unequivocally stated. As far as my limited Chinese allows, I think the first mention in the *Su Wen* of pulse diagnosis is at the very end of Chapter 4:

> "Therefore, those who are truly good at taking the pulse will examine the five viscera and six bowels with great care in order to determine their manifestations... The physicians should

---

5 Pulse diagnosis by various methods is discussed (not an exhaustive list) in *Sù Wèn* chapters 5, 7, 9, 10, 13, 15, 17, 18, 19, 20, 21, 23, 40, 67, and 74. The same topic is addressed in *Líng Shū* chapters 3, 4, 9, 10, and 48. Because this source of pulse teachings in the *Nei Jing* is so extensive, I will only discuss a limited selection from among them.

6 Specific pulse qualities mentioned by Chunyu Yi in the *Shi Ji* (c.94 BCE) included wiry (xian), tight (jin), rapid (shuo), big (da), small (xiao), replete (shi), deep (shen), weak (ruo), hard (jian), even (ping), urgent (ji), scattered (sun), intermittent (dai), slippery (hua), and choppy (se). It seems obvious that these references have nothing to do with the method of comparing radial and carotid artery pulses, but are rather very similar to the descriptions of pulse qualities that have survived into the present in the practice of radial artery pulse diagnosis at the wrist. On the other hand, Liào Píng 廖平 (1851–1914?) wrote, "Since the times (479–557 CE) of Ch'I (齊) and Liang (梁) it was no longer a matter of course to touch the throat or feet of women for diagnosis. Hence this method (of pulse diagnosis at the wrist) was established so that (physicians could continue) to earn their livelihood" (cited in Unschuld 1986, p.29).

> master such important things and commit them to memory without error, and then, they should teach such things to the right and capable persons only..." (Lu 1978, p.29, *Su Wen* 4)

From this introductory passage, I infer that the authors believed that the details of the actual practice of pulse diagnosis were not appropriate to share with just anyone who had access to the writings, but rather were properly part of the oral lineage of master/disciple transmission characteristic of that age. Such a conclusion would explain the absence of clear standards for radial pulse diagnosis in this foundational text, without contradicting its fundamental importance. In the following chapter 5 of *Su Wen*, however, I believe that one can see the authors' assumption that their general remarks on pulse diagnosis referred specifically to examination of the pulses of the radial artery at the wrists:

> "Those who know well how to diagnose, they inspect the color and press the vessels. First they distinguish yin and yang. They investigate what is clear and turbid and know the section... *They press at the foot long section and at the inch (chǐ cùn)*, they observe (whether the movement in the vessels) is in the surface or in the depth, smooth or rough, and they know the location where the disease has emerged." (Unschuld and Tessenow 2011, pp.121–122, *Su Wen* 5)

In order to correctly understand this passage, one must be clear about the reference to "the foot long section and the inch" (chǐ cùn 尺寸), as these technical terms will appear again throughout the corpus of texts on pulse diagnosis. What I would like to emphasize here is that this initial discussion of the pulse clearly does not refer to comparisons of the radial and carotid pulses, a method that, while discussed more fully in other chapters of the *Nei Jing*[7] was neither mentioned nor implied until later chapters of the *Su Wen*. Various interpretations of the meanings of chǐ cùn will be mentioned in my discussion of the *Nan Jing*, but for clarity's sake I will simply translate chǐ as the section of the radial artery at the wrist proximal to the styloid process of the radius, and cùn as the section of the radial artery at the wrist distal to the styloid process of the radius. Another group of terms for this diagnostic region of the radial artery at the wrist, which appears in the *Su Wen*, includes cùn kǒu 寸口 (meaning inch mouth or inch opening), mài kǒu 脈口 (meaning vessel or pulse mouth or opening) and qì kǒu 氣口 (meaning qi mouth or opening). For example, *Su Wen* chapter 11 asks:

> "How comes that only (the movement in the vessels that can be felt at) the qi opening is ruled by the five depots?"

Wang Bing, the editor of our received copy of the *Su Wen*, glossed this passage as follows:

> "the qi opening is the inch opening, another name is vessel opening… In all cases (the information) is taken from (a location) one inch behind the fish-line (at the wrist). This, then is the inch opening." (Unschuld and Tessenow 2011, p.207, footnote 18)

In the next chapter I will return to the importance of Wang's identification of the inch opening as being located one inch proximal to the wrist crease, which is borne out by the received text of chapter 2 of the *Ling Shu*. My impression is that all the

---

7 *Su Wen* chapters 4 and 5 appear to be discussions of radial pulse diagnosis. The first brief appearance of comparing carotid and radial pulses is found in chapter 6, and then elaborated in chapter 7. For a more detailed analysis, see my discussion of the *Ling Shu* in Chapter 5 of the present text.

various terms for this region, cited above, simply refer to the traditional area for radial pulse examination, from the wrist crease past the styloid process, in a manner to allow the index, middle, and ring fingers of the examiner to lie adjacent to each other. The important point here for now is that all these mentions in the *Su Wen*, of places to examine the pulse, are strictly talking about the radial artery in the vicinity of the styloid process of the radius. Thus it seems clear to me that radial pulse diagnosis was well recognized, and probably considered the chief method of pulse diagnosis by the authors of the *Su Wen*.

This point of view is important to keep in mind when one encounters descriptions of the different pulse qualities that resonate with the different categories discussed in the *Nei Jing*, whether they be yīn yáng, wǔ xíng, mài or zàng fǔ. Ironically, however, there is only one passage in the whole of the *Nei Jing* where a presentation is given of the location along the radial artery for examining the pulses associated with the zàng fǔ and their corresponding meridians, and I believe this crucial passage has been misinterpreted by translators (Unschuld and Tessenow 2011, pp.296–297).

For example, chapter 17 has been translated as follows:

> "The exterior of the foot long section serves to examine the kidneys; the interior of the foot long section serves to examine the abdomen. On the central instep on the left, the exterior serves to examine the liver; the interior serves to examine the diaphragm. On the right, the exterior serves to examine the stomach; the interior serves to examine the spleen. On the upper instep on the right, the exterior serves to examine the lung; the interior serves to examine the chest center. On the left, the exterior serves to examine the heart; the interior serves to examine the dan zhong." (Unschuld and Tessenow 2011, pp.296–297)

This passage is obfuscated by the translation of fū (附) as "instep." Unschuld and Tessenow explained this passage as probably unrelated to pulse diagnosis thus: "It remains unclear whether the diagnostic technique outlined in these paragraphs refers to an examination of pulses, or to an inspection of the condition of the skin. The latter possibility appears plausible in view of the distance of the 'central instep' region from the wrists" (Unschuld and Tessenow 2011, p.296, footnote 96). Actually, it is not plausible once we adopt a more appropriate translation for fū (附). If we look up this character in Mathews' dictionary, we find it listed as #1924, and defined as "to attach, to be close to." Applying "close to" or "next to" to this passage leaves us with a description of the traditional pulse associations on left and right sides of the three positions at the wrist, namely cùn 寸, guān 關, and chǐ 尺. Guān is in the middle ("central"), cùn is "upper" (next to), and chǐ is lower (next to, corresponding to "the foot long section"). Returning to the quoted passage from *Su Wen* 17, we find that it is bookended by discussions of the pulse, which practically ensures the accuracy of my interpretation. The prior section begins:

> "If it is verified that the movement in the vessels is diminished, and that the complexion is not lost, it is a new disease." (Unschuld and Tessenow 2011, p.294)

And the following section begins:

> When (the movement in the vessels) is rough and big, the yin is insufficient and the yang has surplus." (Unschuld and Tessenow 2011, p.297)

One more excerpt, from later in the *Su Wen*, solidifies the argument that radial pulse examination was regarded by its authors as an independent, if not the primary, method of pulse diagnosis, without any comparison implied between it and the carotid pulse:

"To treat an illness while disregarding its beginning, without knowing if there is anxiety and suffering, without knowing if food and drink fail to be moderate, without knowing if the life habits are excessive, without knowing if [the patient] may have been injured by poison, to not inquire about these first, but instead abruptly grasp cùn kǒu, how can the illness be correctly addressed?"[8]

8 *Su Wen* chapter 78, translation by Malomlus Paa'ayat, and posted on "Scholars of Chinese Medicine," a Facebook chat group, 8 May 2016.

Chapter 5

Líng Shū 靈樞

SPIRITUAL PIVOT

(a) (b)

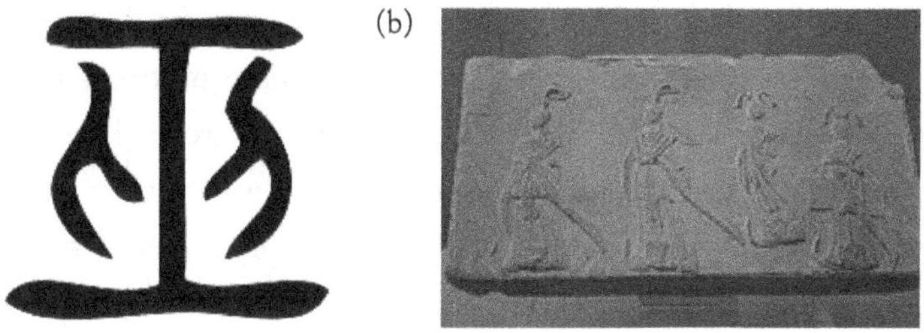

Figure 5.1 Ancient Chinese shamans[1]
Source: Professor Gary Lee Todd

---

1 The top image is the Seal script character for "wu 巫," who were female shamans that had the power to invoke the spirits from Heaven to alter events on Earth. The first Chinese dictionary of characters, the (121 CE) Shuowen Jiezi defines wu as zhu 祝 "sacrifice; prayer master; invoker; priest" (祝也 女能以舞降神者也 象从工 两人舞形, tr. Hopkins 1920, p.432) and analyzes the Seal graph, "An Invoker. A woman who can serve the Invisible, and by posturing bring down the spirits." This Seal graph for wu is interpreted as showing "the 工 work of two dancing figures set to each other—a shamanistic dance" (Karlgren 1923, p.363). Their power is embodied in the character "ling 靈," which incorporates the pictograph of the "wu." Ling expresses the efficacy of the "shen 神," both terms commonly translated into English as spirit or spiritual. The bottom image is a Han dynasty ceramic tile depicting dancing wu and their attendants. Images: https://en.wikipedia.org/wiki/Wu_(shaman). *In the Footsteps of the Yellow Emperor* (Eckman 2007) recounts the contemporary report of an Asian shamanic ritual in Los Angeles in 1977 that was performed after 100 days of drought. Following the ceremony, a cloudburst occurred within hours (Eckman 2007, pp.42–43). Ling is character 4071 in Mathews' dictionary.

The *Ling Shu* comprises the second half of *The Yellow Emperor's Inner Classic* (*Huángdì Nèijīng* 黃帝內經). Líng 靈, which I've translated as "spiritual," depicts two shamans exerting their spiritual power to invoke Heaven to produce rainfall. Some of the other meanings this character can provide include the ideas of quickness and efficacy.[2] Quickness should remind us of the character yìng 應 used in referring to resonance, so the combination of quickness and efficacy aptly serves to communicate the nature of this text, which has also been named *Zhen Jing* 針經 *The Classic of Acupuncture*. One of the most remarkable things about acupuncture, in my experience, is its virtually instantaneous effect on both signs and symptoms (pulse and color changes being the most noticeable, but pain and other subjective manifestations sometimes respond equally rapidly) when the treatment points are well selected.[3] The use of the character líng reminds us, however, that we are dealing with effects emanating from the non-material realm, so traditional acupuncture is best understood from the viewpoint of Eastern rather than Western scientific premises, but the authors of the *Ling Shu* did not expect acupuncture practitioners to actually be shamans. Rather, one simply needs to be able to wield the power inherent in the natural operation of resonant relationships, and the *Ling Shu* provides us with some of the basic knowledge needed to carry such theory into practice.[4]

2 Mathews (1979, 4071). Yabla gives "quick" as the first definition and "efficacious" as the third, with "spirit" as the sixth! See https://chinese.yabla.com/chinese-english-pinyin-dictionary.php?define=靈.

3 While some effects of acupuncture demonstrate this remarkable rapidity, I am not asserting that rapidity of effect is a necessary response to good acupuncture treatment. The question of how fast results may be expected and how long to leave the needles is an entirely separate topic, with many diverse opinions.

4 I disagree with the position expressed by Paul Unschuld in his 2016 translation of the *Ling Shu*, despite the tremendous service he has done in making this classic more accessible to English readers. His introduction on page 1 states, "It is likewise unknown who ultimately gave the work the title *Ling Shu*, or the '*Numinous Pivot*,' which bears no relation to the content of this text, marked

The topic I would like to examine in this chapter is the particular method of pulse diagnosis, and its implications for treatment, which received the most explicit, systematic, and thorough presentation in several chapters of the *Nei Jing*. I'm referring to the rén yíng cùn kǒu 人迎寸口 (hereafter denoted as RYCK) method that compares the pulses in the neck to those at the wrist. I'll preface my remarks by pointing out that RYCK diagnosis is not even mentioned in the contemporary TCM texts that I have read, and that it is certainly a practice used only by a small minority of acupuncturists worldwide. I have been curious about this circumstance for a long time, and will try to account for it by re-examining its textual basis, but in order to buck the tide of orthodox interpretations, I hypothesize that from the earliest times, commentators have simply been repeating what was already written, rather than critically examining the text in light of both clinical results and linguistic analysis.

The first mention in the *Nei Jing* of pulse diagnosis by the method of comparing the carotid and radial pulses occurs in *Su*

as it is by secular reasoning." The mistake I believe Unschuld is making is confusing secularism with materialism. While the text does not resort to gods or ancestors as the perpetrators of human illnesses, it repeatedly states that effective treatment starts from dealing with the afflicted individual's spirit (shén 神). Both shén and *líng* are aspects of, and are translated by, the same word, spirit, and both terms appear in the traditional names of acupuncture points. As early as chapter 1, *Ling Shu* states (in Unschuld's translation), "Unrefined (practitioners) guard the physical appearance. Outstanding (practitioners) guard the spirit." The text continues, "The unrefined (practitioners) guard the trigger. Outstanding (practitioners) guard the (inner) mechanism. The motion of the mechanism never leaves the enclosed empty space. The mechanism in the enclosed empty space is clear, calm and subtle." Does this passage not remind the reader of the progressive descriptions of reality from the *Yi Jing* (wú jí becomes tài jí) to the discussion of gǎn yìng in *Huai Nan Zi*? These metaphysical concepts are essential to understanding the meaning of the *Ling Shu*, both title and text.

Wen chapters 7 and 9,[5] but it is only elaborated into a doctrine for constructing a set of corresponding acupuncture treatments in *Ling Shu* chapter 9. I first took a class on this method taught by Doeki Ogura in Tokyo in 1982, but because some of his claims seemed contrary to my experience,[6] I put away my notes, and didn't revisit them until recently. In the intervening time, I also studied this method under the tutelage of Tae Woo Yoo, the originator of Korean Hand Acupuncture, whose textbook I edited. I previously wrote that my experience in applying this methodology, as taught to me in different ways by both these Japanese and Korean lineage masters,[7] was unreliable, and that I thought either it was an inaccurate method, or that my understanding of how to apply this method of diagnosis needed correction. I suspected that the latter possibility was the correct explanation because it seemed highly unlikely to me that the one method of pulse diagnosis that was most clearly and repeatedly described in the *Nei Jing* would be groundless.

---

5 Unschuld and Tessenow (2011, p.139): "By differentiating at the yang, one knows the location of the disease. By differentiating at the yin, one knows the times of death and survival. (The three yang are at the head; the three yin are at the hands.)" In footnote 8, Wang Bing interprets this passage thus: "'Head' is to say man's facing (ren ying); 'hands' is to say qi opening. The two correspond to each other. If the (movement in the) vessels is equally big or small (at both these locations), as if a rope of equal diameter were pulled (through both locations), one speaks of a healthy person."

6 First, he claimed that a healthy pulse is characterized by the carotid being three times wider than the radial, whereas my experience is that when a person is healthy, these pulse widths are equal (see Wang Bing's commentary in the previous footnote). Second, he claimed that the distinction between whether the hand or foot branch of the Great Meridian is involved depends only on pulse rate (80 beats per minute or more indicating the hand branch, less than 80 indicating the foot branch). My experience indicates that this is not always clinically accurate.

7 *The Compleat Acupuncturist* (Eckman 2014) describes my inability to successfully apply this diagnostic technique.

I asked my colleagues who had good results using this method for guidance in a professional online forum, and was not surprised to find that there were a wide variety of interpretations, especially about the correct location for palpating the radial pulse at cùn kǒu. Tae Woo Yoo had indicated that the correct location for cùn kǒu was at the wrist crease where the acupuncture point LU 9 is located, and as I had studied with him for a number of years, that was how I always carried out the examination; but some practitioners pointed out that, in their training, cùn kǒu was located where the pulse is normally the strongest in the vicinity of the wrist, namely at the crest of the styloid process.[8] As soon as I began using this location, I found that this method of pulse diagnosis was clinically quite useful, but still didn't exactly match the descriptions in the available English translations of the *Nei Jing*. Therefore I attempted my own translation of *Su Wen* chapter 9 to see if it could be interpreted in a way that correlated with my clinical observations, which I will explain shortly. Needless to say, the following translation (admittedly by an amateur linguist) differs significantly from any of those I have seen published in English:[9]

---

8 Personal communication (2016) from Ed Antkowiak: "I was trained to use this method at the Kototama Institute back in the early 80s, in Santa Fe. In Japanese Medicine, it is called Jingei diagnosis (Jin Gei being the Japanese pronunciation of Ren Ying). I have been using it for 32 years. We were also trained to use the styloid location—to position the middle finger. Then, placing the index and ring fingers on the corresponding pulses distal and proximal, finding the strongest position at all three, comparing them to the carotid pulse. Cidian defines cùn kǒu thus: "From the thenar supreme bone, but the line one inch, which is called Cunkou." "TCM pulse": "when the Chinese medicine doctor… hand on the pulse with three fingers on both hands…forearm radial artery, this area is called 'Cunkou'." See http://cidian.xpcha.com/cadg6bzh3hx.html.

9 This passage is reproduced here so that the reader, if conversant with traditional Chinese characters, can follow my reasoning regarding its interpretation: 故人迎一盛病在少陽, 二盛病在太陽, 三盛病在陽明, 四盛上為格陽. 寸口一盛病在厥陰, 二盛病在少陰, 三盛病在太陰, 四盛已上為關陰. 人迎與寸口俱盛四倍已上為關格, 關格之脈赢, 不能極於天地之精氣, 則死矣.

> Thus rén yíng one (measure, and) vigorous (compared to cùn kǒu means) illness is (in) shao yang, two (measures and) vigorous (compared to cùn kǒu means) illness is (in) tai yang, three (measures and) vigorous (compared to cùn kǒu means) illness is (in) yang ming, four (measures and) vigorous (compared to cùn kǒu means the illness) has progressed to[10] obstructed yang. Cùn kǒu one (measure, and) vigorous (compared to rén yíng means) illness is (in) jue yin, two (measures and) vigorous (compared to rén yíng means) illness is (in) shao yin, three (measures and) vigorous (compared to rén yíng means) illness is (in) tai yin, four (measures and) vigorous (compared to rén yíng means the illness) has progressed to closed yin. Rén yíng together with cùn kǒu (both) entirely vigorous four-fold (bèi) (compared to normal, then the illness) has progressed to closed (yin and) obstructed (yang). Closed (and) obstructed, one's pulse (mài) overcomes one's vitality (jīng qì), (which is) limited (by the contributions of) Heaven and Earth (and so one will) die.

The first thing I would like to point out about this passage is that there is a perfectly good classical Chinese character, 倍 (bèi), that can be translated as times or -fold (as in two-fold, three-fold, etc.) In fact, this character is used in the final section of the quoted excerpt, but what is most interesting is that it doesn't appear in any of the sentences that refer to the proportions between the rén yíng

10 https://chinese.yabla.com/chinese-english-pinyin-dictionary.php?define=上 gives as one definition of shang: "to go up" which in this case would mean "to progress to." In the context of the whole passage, the usual translation of upper or above makes no clinical sense to me, especially as the parallel term for cùn kǒu four vigorous is also shang. Unschuld simply leaves shang untranslated in this sentence, rendering the text as "yin closure," but why would that also be upper or above? The text is clearly pointing to the seriousness of an illness with such pulse findings, so "progress to" is the only interpretation that appears to have a clear clinical meaning.

and cùn kǒu pulses. For some reason, however, all the translations I have seen interpret 一盛 (one vigorous or flourishing) as twice, 二盛 (two vigorous), as three times, and so on, an interpretation that one would expect to have been expressed using the character bèi. I have chosen the word "measure(s)" as a placeholder only. What I noticed in my patients was that, if I used the proper locations for palpating the pulses (a subject I will address next), then those with Yang Ming imbalances showed carotid pulses that were not just three times (rather than four times) bigger (and stronger) than the radial pulses, but also felt as though they had three components: a center plus an additional impulse both radially and ulnarly. Since I don't know whether the more significant finding is the relative size or the presence of different numbers of component parts, I am using "measure(s)" to allow for either possibility. It is my impression that this pulse finding is more consistent than feeling the carotid pulse to be four times as big as the radial pulse, which has been the opinion of all the translations and commentaries I have read.

Similarly, those with tai yang imbalances showed carotid pulses that were not just two times (rather than three times) bigger than the radial pulses, but also felt as though they had two components: a center plus an additional impulse either medially or laterally. With shao yang imbalances, the carotid pulse was slightly bigger than the radial pulse, but by much less than a two-to-one ratio, and the carotid pulse had only one central impulse. The exact opposite presentation appeared in my patients with tai yin, shao yin, and jue yin imbalances: now it was the radial pulse that was both bigger (vigorous) and had either three, two, or one component(s). From these findings I decided that my translation was an accurate one. It was only after noticing these clinical correlations in my own practice that I rediscovered a pamphlet describing the Japanese RYCK tradition (Van Meter 2007), and revisited my notes from my 1982 class with Master Ogura. To my great surprise, Ogura had come to exactly the same conclusion about the meaning of the *Su Wen* passage as I had![11] Van Meter's pamphlet describes the shao yang pulse ratio (RYCK) as "almost even: just a little wider in the carotid artery than the radial artery." In order to indicate this slight difference in widths, he gives it a numerical ratio of 1.5 to 1 (which I have adjusted to 1.25 to 1 in order to more accurately reflect what I feel), but in all other respects his ratio interpretations match mine exactly, as shown in Table 5.1.

This leaves me to speculate on what the three, two, and one part impulses might represent. Throughout the classics there are references to the three yang and three yin energies (for want of a better English term), so it seems logical to me to ascribe this finding to a manifestation of the presence of these yin and yang component energies.[12] *Su Wen* chapter 7 uses the terminology of

11 Doeki Ogura (1899–1983) was the lineage founder of the Jingei tradition in Japan. When I studied with him in 1982, the year before he passed away, he had already been using RYCK diagnosis for over 50 years. Among his disciples were Yoshi Ikeda, who taught Van Meter, and Mikoto Masahilo Nakazono (1918–1994), who founded the Kototama Institute in Santa Fe, NM. My lecture notes indicate that Ogura was quite emphatic that the cùn kǒu location on the wrist was at the guan position, right at the crest of the styloid, one inch from the base of the thumb.

12 As stated, the first mention in the *Nei Jing* of pulse diagnosis by comparing carotid and radial arteries occurs in *Su Wen* chapter 7. Immediately preceding, in chapter 6, the *Su Wen* first introduced the notion of the three yang and three yin *mài* and their functions in terms of opening, closing and pivoting. At the same time, chapter 6 can be interpreted as discussing three components of yang qi that together make one yang, and three components of yin qi that together make one yin: "(These) three (yang) conduits cannot lose each other. If they beat, but not at the surface, this is called 'one yang'... These three yin conduits cannot lose each other. If they beat, but not in the depth, this is called 'one yin'." Wang Bing explains (Unschuld and Tessenow 2011, chapter 6, footnotes 26 and 36), "When the arrival of the (qi in the) three (yang) conduits strikes the fingers of one's hand without there being any difference in their being light or heavy, then one is justified to speak of the qi of one yang. The (three yang conduits) do no longer send three (distinguishable) yang (qi) to

"first yang, second yang, third yang, first yin, second yin, third yin."[13] I have not carried this speculation any further in terms of the arrivals of these specific energies (a common expression in the classics), but hope that it will be possible to do so in the future.

Regardless of whether or not further experience might support comparisons of size between the neck and wrist pulses as more reliable than the presence of palpably distinct components, I'm convinced that the quoted passage is best interpreted as referring to ratios of 1:1, 2:1, and 3:1 rather than the usual teachings of 2:1, 3:1, and 4:1. Before examining the question of locations for palpating RYCK, I should point out that this diagnostic method is focused on the present pattern of imbalances, not the individual's original constitution, although in many of the patients I have examined, the present condition reflects the constitutional imbalance, and so it often shows the corresponding pattern in RYCK diagnosis. I have found in my practice that the left-sided RYCK pulse ratios correspond to the imbalances located along the circuit of the principal meridians, while the right-sided pulse

---

move down… When all the conduit qi arrive in full accord, without there being any differences of (movements) at the surface or in the depth, then they can be said to be the qi of one single yin" (Unschuld and Tessenow 2011, pp.132–135). My tentative interpretation of Wang's remarks is that a healthy pulse should feel like it has only one component, applicable to both carotid and radial locations. Thus, finding several components in one of these pulses is evidence that a pathophysiological state exists, and needs rectifying (by acupuncture treatment, as described in detail in the subsequent passage in *Ling Shu* chapter 9).

13 The commentaries cited in the footnotes to Unschuld's translation identify these as: first yang = shao yang, second yang = yang ming, third yang = tai yang, first yin = jue yin, second yin = shao yin, third yin = tai yin. This model is found in other places in the *Nei Jing*, and is essentially depicting the same model as presented in the *Shang Han Lun*, if understood in the way I have described in *The Book of Changes in Traditional Oriental Medicine* (Eckman 1988).

ratios correspond to the Organ system imbalances.[14] In cases where these ratios are not distinctly one-to-one on the left side, it has been my experience that an entry/exit block exists between a pair of principal meridians, and that treating the respective entry and exit points is needed before any further balancing of the Organ systems (zàng fŭ).[15] These conclusions are supported

14 I am grateful to Ian Harp for suggesting the difference in laterality of the RYCK pulses, and the putative relationship of RYCK pulses to the meridians as opposed to the deeper functions of the zàng fŭ as elaborated in the following footnote.

15 There appear to be two ways the human organism maintains homeostatic balance through the medium of qì. The first is via the mutual influence of the Organ systems (zàng fŭ) as seen in the shēng and kè cycle relationships. This resembles a kind of radiant, or non-localized, influence of the various forms of qì. The second is via the continuous flow of qì along the pathways of the 12 principal meridians, which is a more linear and localized manifestation of qì flow. One way of visualizing this dichotomy is by its analogy to a simple room heater: the first mechanism corresponds to the radiation of heat, while the second corresponds to the conduction of heat (exemplified by accidentally touching the radiator). Worsley's teacher, Lavier, transmitted to him (Lavier 1966, pp.91–92) the terminology of the meridian flow being called the "wèi" circulation, and the Five Element interactions being called the "yíng" circulation (which Worsley referred to only as the "deep" circulation). It is interesting to speculate on whether these two aspects of qì represent the same phenomena as are referred to in the canonical references to wèi and yíng qì. If so, one can envision the mutual influence of these two aspects of qì dynamics as the explanation for the change in what the RYCK pulses show when there is an entry/exit block present. My current hypothesis of how the qì dynamic manifests in the pulse is as follows. The left RYCK pulses reflect the state or functionality of the meridian system (linear, conduction analogy), and abnormalities in these RYCK pulses are best treated by clearing entry/exit blocks on the principal meridians. The right RYCK pulses reflect the state or functioning of the zàng fŭ systems (non-linear, radiation analogy), whose imbalances are best treated by any method that addresses the wŭxíng 五行 relationships of the zàng fŭ in order to normalize them. Traditionally, the left side is yang and the right side is yin, so we can understand these differences of laterality (meridians are yang with respect to the Organs) as following basic yin yang theory. The cùn 寸, guan 關, and chǐ 尺 pulses at the wrist predominantly reflect the wŭ xíng relationships of the zàng fŭ, although they may secondarily be affected by blocks along the principal meridians. Thus both RYCK pulse examination and cùn 寸, guan 關,

by several types of evidence, the first being the observation that RYCK pulses change after treatment from their initial state of imbalance to one of equality, or balance, providing the treatment was correctly chosen and applied. Also, the quotation states that when the ratio of pulses has progressed to four-to-one, a state of obstruction or closure has occurred. Progression implies an evolving disease process, not a constitutional manifestation.

Not all commentators are even in agreement that RYCK diagnosis refers to comparisons of the carotid and radial pulses. The paired terms rén yíng and cùn kǒu are a good example of the need to use context when interpreting the meaning of classical Chinese texts. In the *Nei Jing* it seems clear that in applying this pair of terms to pulse diagnosis, the meaning is a comparison of the carotid and radial arteries. The same pair of terms is apparently used in other texts to refer to the left radial pulse as rén yíng and the right radial pulse as cùn kǒu, possibly occurring as early as in Difficulty 23 of the *Nan Jing*, where it says, "In the morning the qi begins its passage at cùn kǒu and rén yíng, at the yin and yang." As we will see in Chapter 6 on the *Nan Jing*, that text was clear that all the qi (both yin and yang) begins and ends its circulation at the "inch opening" of the wrist, so rén yíng would appear to mean the left radial pulse in the quoted passage; but as this is the only chapter in the *Nan Jing* to mention rén yíng, its interpretation must remain an open question. Note the reversed order of these two terms, however, perhaps indicating a change in context from that in the *Nei Jing*. Hua Shou 滑壽 (c.1340, quoted in Unschuld 1986, pp.89 and 294) attributed this second set of meanings for

and chǐ 尺 pulse examination can each provide information about the coupled phenomena of meridian and Organ systems, but using them together provides the most complete and cross-validated information. Personally, I have confirmed these findings by additionally incorporating the Ayurvedic pulse diagnostic interpretations that I described in *The Compleat Acupuncturist* (Eckman 2014), but that is unfortunately too large a topic to reprise here.

rén yíng and cùn kǒu (more exactly qì kǒu, a synonym) to Wang Shuhe (王叔和 210–285 CE) in his text, the *Mai Jing*, an opinion shared by Omura (1982, p.218). This second meaning of these two terms is generally discredited as being applicable to RYCK diagnosis. It was, however, taught in this misunderstood fashion in the Western acupuncture community, based on Nguyen Van Nghi's translation of the *Ling Shu*: "According to the translation of Van Nghi, Cun Kou is the right radial artery and Ren Ying is the left radial artery."[16]

TABLE 5.1 RÉN YÍNG/CÙN KǑU DIAGNOSIS

Rén yíng/cùn kǒu ratio	*Pulse quality*	*Imbalance diagnosis*
1.25/1	Normal	Foot Shao Yang (GB Excess)
1.25/1	Bustling (zào 躁)	Hand Shao Yang (TH Excess)
2/1	Normal	Foot Tai Yang (UB Excess)
2/1	Bustling (zào 躁)	Hand Tai Yang (SI Excess)
3/1	Normal	Foot Yang Ming (ST Excess)
3/1	Bustling (zào 躁)	Hand Yang Ming (LI Excess)
4/1		Obstructed Yang
1/1.25	Normal	Foot Jue Yin (LV Excess)
1/1.25	Bustling (zào 躁)	Hand Jue Yin (PE Excess)
1/2	Normal	Foot Shao Yin (KI Excess)

16 www.ebramec.com.br/uploads/downloads/radial-carotida_bases%20e%20aplicacoes_neijing.pdf.

1/2	Bustling (zào 躁)	Hand Shao Yin (HE Excess)
1/3	Normal	Foot Tai Yin (SP Excess)
1/3	Bustling (zào 躁)	Hand Tai Yin (LU Excess)
1/4		Closed Yin
4/4		Closed Yin and Obstructed Yang

The next issue is concerned with the locations of rén yíng and cùn kǒu along the carotid and radial arteries in RYCK diagnosis. Rén yíng is the Chinese name of the acupuncture point ST 9, located on the neck where the carotid artery can be felt pulsating. Literally it means "man's forging ahead."[17] There are two reasons I find this translation of the point name preferable to that commonly found. The choice of "man's" here I believe is an indication that men and women have different anatomy in this location (i.e., a prominent Adam's Apple in men, which is generally absent in women). As for "forging ahead," this is an extremely yang concept, and rén yíng is the site where the qi of the yang meridians manifests and is evaluated in RYCK diagnosis. Thus man's forging ahead is a fitting description, both structurally and functionally.[18] In practice, however, it is not always found at the classical site given for ST 9

17 人: Mathews 1979, 3097; 迎: Mathews 1979, 7473. The more common translation is "man's welcome." Although I understand the possible interpretation of such a name as having a spirit level connotation in the context of the Worsley tradition of using the Windows of the Sky (of which ST 9 is a member), it makes little sense to me in other contexts. Therefore I am choosing one translation of yíng provided by yabla: https://chinese.yabla.com/chinese-english-pinyin-dictionary.php?define=迎.

18 Yíng could also be translated as "meeting," which could convey the functional concept of the convergence of yang, but not the structural analogy with the Adam's Apple. The same reasoning applies to translating yíng as prognosis (as in Ellis *et al.* 1989).

(one and a half inches on either side of the midline), but might be more lateral, in the vicinity of LI 17, or wherever the carotid pulse is felt. For RYCK diagnosis, it is the pulsating place in males on the same vertical level as the crest of the Adam's Apple.[19] Following the teachings of my Korean mentor, Tae Woo Yoo, I find that the location for palpating rén yíng in women is usually somewhat lower, at the level of the cricothyroid membrane, but this may not be the case if they have a male pattern thyroid cartilage (Adam's Apple), in which case that is the location to use. It is not difficult to find a rationale for these varied locations: above and distal (from the Heart) are yang (as is male), below and proximal (towards the Heart) are yin (as is female) displaying the resonance of yin and yang typical of all phenomena.

I have already introduced the controversy regarding the location of cùn kǒu. An important thing to keep in mind here, as with all issues in Chinese medicine, is the previous assertion that terms are not absolute in their meanings, but are relative to the context in which they are being used. Sometimes they denote one possible meaning, sometimes a different possible meaning, and often leave multiple possible interpretations as a kind of "poetic" image, characteristic of classical Chinese literature. This situation has advantages in its emphasis on the interconnectedness of nature, expressed in resonance theory, but it can be a problem when one needs to choose the appropriate location to examine a pulse, for example cùn kǒu in this case. *Ling Shu* chapter 2 gives what I consider to be a clearly specified location for cùn kǒu in its presentation of the five shu points (wǔ shū xué) on the Lung

19 Ogura used a different criterion for locating the neck pulse: he recommended feeling for the place on the carotid artery that was the widest. Perhaps this difference in methodology is responsible for his observation that the vast majority of people he examined had carotid pulses that were three times wider than their radial pulses, which in turn led him to conclude that this yang ming pattern represented the healthy state.

meridian.[20] It describes the fourth shu point from the tip of the thumb (LU 8, Jing Qu 經渠) as located at the center of cùn kǒu, which implies that cùn kǒu covers an unspecified area of the wrist normally palpated in pulse diagnosis, with the point LU 8 at its center, at the crest of the styloid, one cun proximal to LU 9.[21] There should be no doubt, however, that cùn kǒu can be used as a general term to include the whole area of the radial artery near the wrist where practitioners of Chinese medicine typically examine

---

20 歧伯曰: 請言其次也. 肺出於少商, 少商者, 手大指端內側也, 為井木; 溜于魚際, 魚際者, 手魚也, 為滎; 注于太淵, 太淵魚後一寸陷者中也, 為俞; 行於經渠; 經渠寸口中也, 動而不居為經, 入于尺澤, 尺澤肘中之動脈也, 為合. 手太陰經也. http://ctext.org/huangdi-neijing/ling-shu-jing.

21 This passage is translated in Unschuld (2016, pp.54–55). As far as I can determine, there is no definitive statement in the *Nei Jing* describing the specific location of cùn kǒu to use in the chapters pertaining to RYCK diagnosis, so although I will present alternative proposals, in the absence of contrary statements later in the *Ling Shu*, I believe LU 8, at the guan position, is the correct one to choose. For the sake of completeness, it appears that there are three possible interpretations of the cùn kǒu location: at the wrist crease where point LU 9 is located, one inch proximally from there where point LU 8 is located (at the styloid process), and generically the whole distal area of the radial artery near the wrist where the pulse is ordinarily felt in Chinese medicine. My interpretation of cùn kǒu (at least in RYCK diagnosis) as being located at the styloid process of the radius is supported by the philological and historical references I have cited, as well as the clinical findings I have reported. "The character 寸 is an indicative. In the Later Seal Character, it consists of 又 and 一; the former means 'the right hand' and the latter is a sign marking the position on the lower arm about a little longer than an inch away from the wrist. This is the place where a traditional Chinese doctor feels the pulse of a patient. The character 口 has the shape of an open mouth of a man or an animal, hence the primary meaning 'mouth'. Devoid of any stroke in the centre, 口 may also refer to anything with an opening, for example 山口 (mountain pass), 海口 (seaport), 洞口 (mouth of a cave)." www.gxxd.net.cn:1001/date%5CH%5CB3056422.pdf. See also Unschuld and Tessenow (2011, p.207, footnote 18), referencing Wang Bing's location of cùn kǒu at one inch from the wrist crease in *Su Wen* Chapter 11. Wang Bing also commented on *Su Wen* chapter 7 thus: "The qi opening is located one inch behind the fish-line (separating wrist and palm)" as noted in Unschuld and Tessenow (2011, p.139, footnote 8).

the pulses, and in addition may have alternatively specified the pulse felt at the wrist crease in the *Nan Jing* and the *Mai Jing*, to be discussed later.[22]

Finally it is time to discuss the part of *Ling Shu* chapter 9 that motivated me to include it in this treatise. Although the *Ling Shu* does present many dicta about the correct way to practice acupuncture, most of its teachings are either of a general philosophical nature, or else specific recommendations for treating defined pathophysiological states. Chapter 9 is the only one I am aware of that gives a systematic approach to the transitions from examination to diagnosis to method of treatment, to prognosis, applicable to virtually any patient, regardless of their illness (bìng 病) or its current symptomatology.

The first thing this chapter adds is a way to distinguish imbalances in the meridians of the hand branches from those of the foot branches of the same "great meridian" (shao yang, yang ming, tai yang, tai yin, shao yin, or jue yin). A simple distinction is given: the default diagnosis is an imbalance of the foot branch unless a particular pulse quality is present, which is called bustling

22 "There are many pulses in the body, but the place where Chinese doctors take the pulse is called the 'inch mouth' (cùn kǒu). This refers to the radial artery at the styloid processes of the wrists. Chinese doctors have been feeling the pulses diagnostically at this location for at least 2000 years. It is believed that pathological changes in the entire body are reflected in changes in the pulses at this position. In practice, this pulse is first divided into three sections (san bu), the inch, bar, and cubit. The practitioner begins by resting their middle finger directly over the patient's styloid process. This is called the guan or bar position because it separates the other two positions. Then the practitioner's index finger falls into the space between the styloid process and the hypothenar eminence. This is called the cun or inch position because it is one inch wide. The practitioner's ring finger then falls just proximal to their middle finger. This position is called the chi or cubit position because there is one cubit in length between this position and the crook of the elbow." From a Facebook post by Mervin Huang, entitled "Pulse Feeling in Traditional Chinese Medicine," uploaded 25 April 2008.

(zào 躁: Mathews 1979, 6729) a quality that is not found in the standard list of pulse qualities, and is therefore subject to varying interpretations. If the pulse is bustling, then the hand branch of the meridian is imbalanced, otherwise it is the foot branch.[23] My impression is that bustling pulses usually have an "aggressive" quality that might be expressed as being rapid, pounding or sharp in contour, but also feel as if their edges are clearly demarcated, whereas pulses without a bustling quality seem to have edges that fade off almost imperceptibly. Immediately after reprising the RYCK material from *Su Wen* chapter 9, with the additional identification of the foot or hand branch of the meridian that is excessive, *Ling Shu* chapter 9 presents the treatment protocols that are summarized in Table 5.2.[24]

---

23 The Chinese text states: 人迎一盛, 病在足少陽, 一盛而躁, 病在手少陽. 人迎二盛, 病在足太陽, 二盛而躁, 病在手太陽, 人迎三盛, 病在足陽明, 三盛而躁, 病在手陽明. 人迎四盛, 且大且數, 名曰溢陽, 溢陽為外格. 脈口一盛, 病在足厥陰; 厥陰一盛而躁, 在手心主. 脈口二盛, 病在足少陰; 二盛而躁, 在手少陰. 脈口三盛, 病在足太陰; 三盛而躁, 在手太陰. 脈口四盛, 且大且數者, 名曰溢陰. 溢陰為內關, 內關不通, 死不治. 人迎與太陰脈口俱盛四倍以上, 名曰關格. 關格者, 與之短期. Note that mài kǒu (脈口) has replaced cùn kǒu (寸口) in this iteration, showing that the two terms are considered synonyms.

24 As an example of how this material has been translated into English, the following excerpt from Lu (1978, pp.733–734) is quoted. *The reader should keep in mind that I disagree with the translation of the numerical ratios.* "When the pulse in the neck is twice as big as that at the wrist, the little yang of the foot should be sedated, and the decreasing yin of the foot should be toned up. The number of points picked out in sedation therapy should double that in tonification therapy. One treatment should take place each day, and it is also necessary to take the pulse regularly both at the wrist and at the neck in order to determine any change that might have occurred in the conditions of the patient. The points picked out for treatment should be distant from the affected region, and needling should not be stopped until sufficient energy has been induced by the needle to the affected region in order to strike a balance."

TABLE 5.2 SUMMARY OF TREATMENT PROTOCOLS PRESENTED IN *LING SHU* CHAPTER 9

Excess meridian	*First tonify*	*Times punctured*	*Second disperse*	*Times punctured*	*Per day*
GB	LV	1	GB	2	1
TH	PE	1	TH	2	1
UB	KI	1	UB	2	0.5
SI	HE	1	SI	2	0.5
ST	SP	1	ST	2	2
LI	LU	1	LI	2	2
LV	GB	2	LV	1	1
PE	TH	2	PE	1	1
KI	UB	2	KI	1	0.5
HE	SI	2	HE	1	0.5
SP	ST	2	SP	1	2
LU	LI	2	LU	1	2

I believe this passage from *Ling Shu* chapter 9 is very close in spirit to that of the *Nan Jing*, which I will be discussing next. Not only is there an attempt to provide a rational progression from examination to diagnosis and finally to treatment and prognosis, but the points to be treated in every case are the distal points on the indicated meridians. Most of the *Ling Shu* treatment prescriptions select acupuncture points from the whole trajectory of the principal meridians, whereas the focus of the *Nan Jing* shifts to selecting mainly distal points on these meridians, often conceptualized as containing the grouping referred to as the "command points."[25] *Ling Shu* chapter 9 gives specific directions for how to time treatments, not only in terms of the parameters in

25 These include, but are not strictly limited to, the Five Shu Points (also known as the Five Element Points), the Luo or Connecting Points and the Yuan or Source Points.

Table 5.2, but more generally in the advice to treat until the pulses indicate that the imbalanced ascending qi has been harmonized, at which time the needles should be removed.

There are also a number of other controversial topics addressed in *Ling Shu* chapter 9. One commonly hears practitioners of Chinese medicine say that there are no patterns of Kidney Excess, and that the Kidney Meridian should never be dispersed. Table 5.1 clearly refutes this dogma by providing instructions on how to disperse the Kidney when RYCK pulses show a shao yin pattern without bustling pulses. I should mention here that in Korean Hand Acupuncture, as taught by its originator Tae Woo Yoo, one commonly disperses the Kidney when the abdominal presentations indicate it is in excess, and practitioners have had great success using this approach.

Another controversial topic is the question of whether coupled meridians of the same Element should be treated with the same or opposite polarities of stimulation. The Worsley Five Element school teaches that ordinarily both the yin and yang meridians of an imbalanced Element should be treated with the same polarity, that is, either tonification or dispersion. The sole exception is when the pulses indicate an imbalance between these two coupled meridians, a situation that is dealt with by tonifying the luo point of the deficient meridian, but this situation has been a distinctly rare occurrence in my many years of study with Worsley and his lineage followers. *Ling Shu* chapter 9 obviously disagrees with the Worsley approach, as yin and yang coupled meridians are always treated with opposite polarities, as noted in Table 5.2. I believe a partial answer to this apparent conundrum is that there are two different issues that acupuncture treatment addresses when treating coupled meridians of the same Element: the first is the relationship of yin and yang within that Element (addressed in the *Ling Shu*); while the second is the relationship of that Element as a whole to the other four Elements (addressed in the Five Element teachings). Both the first and the second issue need to be addressed in order to be considered optimal treatments, but using just one of these two approaches is still capable of improving the patient's health when used by itself, an interpretation that validates the teachings in both *Ling Shu* chapter 9 and in the Five Element schools. I used the term "partial" deliberately, because it is not just the Worsley school that follows the principle of both meridians of an imbalanced Element typically expressing the same polarity. I will explore this issue in greater detail in discussing the *Nan Jing*, but as a foretaste, I will mention that when we include the different manifestations of qì (both wèi and róng), it is possible to find an interpretation that satisfies both schools of thought: for example, the Lung can have excess róng qì and deficient wèi qì (called Lung yin Excess), at the same time that the Large Intestine will have excess róng qì and deficient wèi qì (called Large Intestine yang Excess). I believe *Ling Shu* chapter 9 begins to examine this topic in its description of the effects of needling at three different depths. The first two depths (superficial and somewhat deeper to deal with yang and yin perverse qi < xié qì 邪氣 >) affect the body's wèi qì 衛氣, while deep needling affects the body's róng qì 榮氣, which is responsible for correcting imbalances in the meridians. I will elaborate on this interpretation in the next chapter; however, I see it as another example of the similarity of thinking between the *Ling Shu* and the *Nan Jing*.

The next controversial topic dealt with in *Ling Shu* chapter 9 is the question of how to differentiate excess from deficient pulses, and I particularly like the answer it gives, as the focus is not merely on theoretical distinctions but rather on the prognostic implications of the changes in the pulses following treatment. The basic question many practitioners struggle with is whether the distinction between excess and deficient pulses is related more to the size or volume of the pulse, as opposed to the quality of the pulse as manifested in its "solidity" or "hollowness." *Ling Shu* chapter 9 clearly indicates that only a change in solidity or hollowness in the desired direction has prognostic value, so that a positive change in this parameter, even if the patient experiences no improvement right after treatment, will result in them experiencing improvement later on. Conversely, if the pulse quality does not change in the expected direction, even if the patient reports feeling better right away, there will be no lasting improvement. The size of the pulse, whether big or small, is, however, not correlated in this passage with prognostic significance.

Finally, *Ling Shu* chapter 9 begins to address the question of the relative amounts of qì and blood in the different meridians. Only one line bears on this topic, but the text says that the reason tai yin and yang ming are best treated twice a day (more often than any of the other meridians) is because the Stomach (which is a yang ming meridian) is the source of nourishment, and therefore has both more blood and more qì to work with. It will be intriguing if this explanation can be expanded to account for the treatment frequency recommended for the other meridians.

Chapter 6

Nán Jīng 難經

THE CLASSIC OF DIFFICULTIES

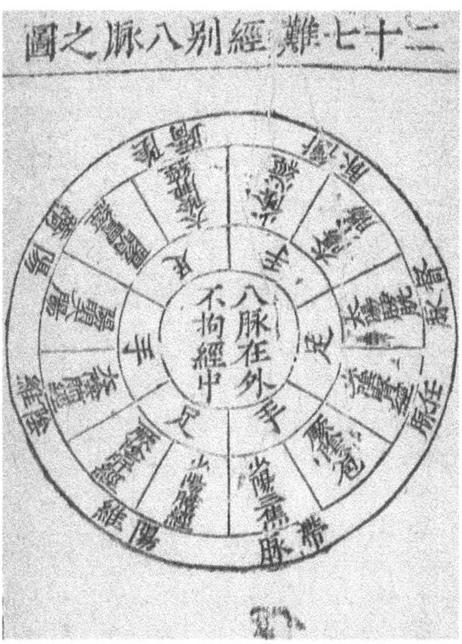

Figure 6.1 Representation of the 12 principal and 8 extraordinary meridians[1]
Source: Wellcome Images

1 From *Tuzhu Nanjing Maijue*, an illustrated compilation of two major classics of Chinese medicine—*Maijue* (Verses on the Pulses) and *Nan Jing* (Classic of 81 Difficulties)—made by Zhang Shixian in the Ming period (1368–1644). This edition, published in 1510, contains specially engraved illustrations. The one pictured is said to refer to the 27th of the "81 Difficulties."

The *Nan Jing* is a text reputed to be from the late Han dynasty (first or second century CE)[2] of unknown authorship (legendarily attributed to Bian Que, c.401–310 BCE) that is usually considered to be a commentary on enigmatic statements made in the *Huángdì Nèijīng*. Since the version of the *Nèijīng* that has survived into the present era (the received text) was compiled and edited by the eleventh-century Imperial Editorial Office (beginning in 1053 CE) and was based considerably on Wang Bing's 762 CE revised version,[3] it is entirely possible that the version of the *Nan Jing* available to us represents a more authentic, or at least less editorialized, version of classical, or even pre-classical, Chinese medical thought.

There are several issues that are discussed in the *Nan Jing* that I wish to explore in this chapter. The first one I have already addressed in the *Journal of Chinese Medicine* (UK) (Eckman 2015), but will mention again here, as it naturally follows up on my earlier presentations regarding radial pulse diagnosis and the meaning of the term cùn kǒu in the *Nei Jing*. Historically, the *Nan Jing* is perhaps the earliest extant text to use the trilogy of cùn 寸,

2 I say "reputed" because there are problems with this orthodox dating. In a personal communication, Dr. Igor Simonov reports that some of the *Nan Jing*'s linguistic expressions were only used in "Old Chinese" as opposed to the later "Classical Chinese" of the Han dynasty. An example he gives is from Difficulty 21 which reads, 非有不病者也 (no have no ill). According to Simonov, after 300 BCE the Classical Chinese way of expressing this double negative would have been 不不 (no no), so the text must have been composed prior to 300 BCE. An additional piece of evidence cited by Simonov is the statement in Difficulty 1, which says that the water clock goes *under* 100 cuts (kè 刻), meaning at that time the Chinese used the *outflow* clepsydra (water clock), in which the level of water *goes down*. The *inflow* clepsydra, based on water *flowing into* the vessel began to be used starting in the Han dynasty (as reported in Needham 1956), implying that Difficulty 1 must have been composed prior to the Han dynasty. Following this logic, the *Nei Jing*'s two component texts were probably of an even earlier date, but were more corrupted by copyists and editors over the long span of time preceding the received edition of 1053 CE.

3 https://en.wikipedia.org/wiki/Huangdi_Neijing.

guān 關, and chǐ 尺, terms it introduces (curiously somewhat late in the received text), but does not explicitly define.[4] I take that situation (the lack of stringent definitions) to be circumstantial evidence supporting a much earlier usage of these three terms as part of radial pulse diagnosis, presumably in lost texts, or merely in oral lineages of transmission. It is hard for me to believe that the first text to use these terms would not have provided clear explanations of where to place one's fingers to correctly examine cùn, guān, and chǐ, unless these terms were already in common usage. Actually, my *JCM* article was written to try to rectify the ongoing absence of any explicit and stringent criteria for locating these pulse positions, not only in the classics, but also in virtually all the subsequent texts on Chinese medicine.

It appears to me that the *Nan Jing*'s explanation of pulse examination is progressively developed in three chapters following a numerological sequence, typical of classical Chinese medical texts. Chapter 1 presents the inch opening (cùn kǒu 寸口) as reflecting all the conduits of the organism ("the great meeting point of the vessels," corresponding, in my opinion, to tài jí 太極),[5] yet without describing its exact location. Since cùn kǒu is a term that was employed repeatedly in the *Nei Jing*, it is understandable that the authors of the *Nan Jing* felt no need to specify its location, but that still leaves the possibility that the authors of these texts used the term differently. If, however, cùn kǒu is the meeting point that reflects all the conduits of the

4 Elisabeth Hsu has written that there are no depictions of pulse-taking procedures in surviving early, or even medieval, Chinese texts, leading to our contemporary situation where different interpretations have been proposed for even the most basic locational reference positions, namely cùn, guān, and chǐ. http://gesnerus.ch/fileadmin/media/pdf/2008_1-2/005-029_Hsu.pdf.

5 Unschuld (1986, pp.82–83 and 89) cites this commentary by Kato Bankei (1784): "The first difficult issue...utilized the image of the original unity (tài jí 太極) before its differentiation (into the categories of yin and yang)."

organism, then the most likely meaning would seem to be the region of the radial artery on the wrist where practitioners place their three fingers to evaluate all the conduits.[6] Chapter 2, however, divides this location (which it now calls chǐ cùn 尺寸, or foot inch, but still referred to as "the great important meeting point of the vessels," previously designated as cùn kǒu) into inch (cùn) and foot (chǐ) sections (reflecting yang and yin respectively). In the case of chǐ cùn, the *Nan Jing* gives a specific location covering 1.9 inches from the wrist crease proximally, and divided into a distal part occupying a length of 0.9 cùn from the wrist crease proximally to the gate (guān 關, which, from its location, must refer to the styloid process), and a proximal part extending another 1 cùn proximally, implying that this crucial area for pulse diagnosis, originally designated as cùn kǒu, covers a length of 1.9 cùn, and since it extends proximally from the wrist crease past the styloid, it cannot refer to the pulse felt at LU 9, but rather must mean the entire region of the radial artery where the pulse is traditionally felt using three fingers.[7] This interpretation is confirmed in chapter 18, which presents the fully developed

6 The discussion of RYCK diagnosis in Chapter 5 strongly supports this location of cùn kǒu (i.e., in the area where practitioners place their three fingers for traditional pulse diagnosis, centered on the styloid process). However, the text does differentiate the "great meeting point (cùn kǒu)" from the "great important meeting point (chǐ cùn)," so it is plausible that these terms indicate different locations from each other, and possibly that the cùn kǒu of the *Nan Jing* has a different connotation than that of the *Nei Jing*, as will be discussed further on in the present text.

7 My interpretation of the meaning of cùn kǒu in the *Nan Jing* is strongly opposed by Simonov, who gives cogent arguments that cùn kǒu must refer specifically to the pulse felt at LU 9. I will be presenting his point of view shortly, as his reasoning is not without merit. He interprets the location of chǐ cùn 尺寸 as being proximal to that of cùn kǒu, and he locates the cùn pulse position at the crest of the styloid process, whereas the conventional interpretation is that the styloid process is actually the location of the guān pulse. One possible source of confusion regarding the location of cùn kǒu in TCM theory might be a result

description of inch (cùn 寸), gate (guān 關) and foot (chǐ 尺) sections, each designating a location where the examiner places his or her fingers, reflecting the differentiated energetics of the Heaven–Man–Earth trilogy as represented in the human organism's 12 conduits.[8] This progression seems to clearly echo *Lao Zi* chapter 42: "Dao produces unity; unity produces duality; duality produces trinity; trinity produces all things."[9]

I like to think of the description of cùn kǒu in chapter 1, which I have just discussed (meaning the place where the practitioner

---

of acupoint LU 9 (太淵 Tàiyuán), Great Abyss, as being designated as the meeting point (會穴 huì xué) of the vessels (first cited in *Nan Jing* chapter 45), which could be interpreted as the *Nan Jing*'s referent for cùn kǒu as the great meeting point of the vessels.

8 Unschuld (1986) chapter 1 states: "The inch opening constitutes the great meeting point of the vessels." Chapter 2 states: "The foot and inch (section) is the great important meeting point of the vessels. From the gate to the foot…is ruled by the yin. From the gate to the fish-line…is ruled by the yang… Hence, the yin comprehended from a one-inch section…the yang comprehended from a 9 fen section… The total length of the foot and inch extends over one inch and nine fen." This passage appears to me to indicate the crest of the styloid as the gate (guān), and in this early description, the gate has no length, it merely separates the foot (chǐ) and inch (cùn) sections of the pulse, which together occupy 1.9 cùn. Hua Shou's gloss states: "The gate is the dividing line formed by the elevated bone behind the palms. It lies behind the inch and in front of the foot as a borderline between the two areas of yin and yang." This preliminary chapter does not describe the finger positions corresponding to cùn, guān, and chi. If any interpretation can be made of this passage, it would appear that the inch both proximal and distal to the crest of the styloid would overlap what is subsequently designated as the location of the guān pulse position. Thus one can see that the meaning of the term "cùn" (as well as the meaning of "guān" and "chǐ") depends on context, and varies in the chapters under discussion. Chapter 18 provides the first differentiation of three sections of the radial pulse for examination: "The vessels appear in three sections; each section has four conduits…" Unschuld (1986, p.257) also notes that Kato Bankei has proposed that the material on cùn, guān and chǐ in chapter 18 should be considered as being chapter 3 (implying that the original text was later rearranged, an interpretation in concordance with my presentation).

9 道生一, 一生二, 二生三, 三生萬物.

places three fingers over a section of the radial artery occupying about two cùn in length) as the exoteric, or conventional, understanding of the opening chapter of this fundamental text on acupuncture practice. However, there is also material in chapter 1 that I think of as esoteric, because I have rarely encountered a practitioner who employed this additional material in clinical practice. I am referring to the presentation of information on the movement of qì 氣 and mài 脈 (pulsation) through the meridians in terms of cycles that are specified in terms of distances, times, and the division of qì 氣 into its dual manifestations as róng 榮 and wèi 衛.[10] Should an alternative to the conventional interpretation of chapter 1 be accepted (as I hope to show to be a credible possibility), it could lead to a radical reinterpretation of the following chapters of the *Nan Jing*. The interpretation I am going to present as a hypothesis for the meaning of this passage in chapter 1, and those that follow, is frankly extremely unorthodox, and it is entirely due to the research of Igor Simonov, who kindly granted me permission to include this material, as he has not as yet written a comprehensive document presenting his research and discoveries.

Before explaining his ideas,[11] I want to make it perfectly clear that my reason for transmitting this material is twofold: first, that each of the implications of his translation of the text leads to a method of examining the pulse that can either validate or reject his conclusions; and second, that I have preliminarily tested

10 From *Nan Jing* 1: 人一呼脈行三寸, 一吸脈行三寸, 呼吸定息, 脈行六寸. 人一日一夜, 凡一萬三千五百息, 脈行五十度, 周於身. 漏水下百刻, 榮衛行陽二十五度, 行陰亦二十五度, 為一周也, 故五十度復會於手太陰. 寸口者, 五藏六府之所終始, 故法取於寸口也. Note that this text uses 榮 róng rather than the later term 營 yíng as the paired term with 衛 wèi qì.

11 To be perfectly clear, this presentation is only my grasp of Simonov's teachings. He might very well think that I am not completely accurate in my understanding of his work.

these pulse findings myself, and by using them have often been led to effective acupuncture treatments. However, my experience with this approach to treatment is a recent area of exploration, and I hope other practitioners will test it out in order to evaluate its clinical reliability. I will not try to cover all the material that Simonov has interpreted (from his theoretical exegeses to the practical use of this information in providing guidance for the practice of acupuncture), and I make no judgment on the validity of any claims of his not presented here; that is something I would leave to anyone who wishes to follow up on this introduction to his work by studying directly with him, an opportunity which I highly recommend, as he is an excellent and most generous teacher.

I think the best way to introduce this interpretation of the *Nan Jing* is by selecting statements from the text, and then presenting the pulse manifestations that Simonov has discovered, which can be interpreted as both reflecting and explaining these statements. From Difficulty 1, I will start with two excerpts that lead to a general statement about the daily cycle of qì in all humans, as reflected in their pulse:

> "Every day and night (24 hours) a person's pulse (reflecting their qi) travels 50 times (during one) circulation through the body..."
>
> "Róng and wèi (qì) travel 25 times through the yang (and) travel 25 times through the yin also. (This) makes one circulation (through the body, so they) circulate 50 times."[12]

The text seems to be saying that something (the circulation of qì through the body) happens in two parts of 25 times each, making a total of 50 parts. These parts are the róng (yíng) qì and

12 The Chinese text reads: 人一日一夜…脈行五十度周於身…榮衛行陽二十五度行陰亦二十五度.為一周也故五十度. The English version is my paraphrasing of Simonov's translation.

the wèi qì, the former traveling through the meridians and the latter outside the meridians. Now, in one day there are 24 hours composed of 1440 minutes. If there are 50 parts to this circulation, then each part should have a duration of exactly 28.8 minutes. Additionally, we know that these parts are róng qì and wèi qì. Róng qì is yin with respect to wèi qì, which is yang. Therefore, if it were possible to feel the pulse exhibiting a movement towards the depth every 28.8 minutes, accompanied by a movement towards the surface every 28.8 minutes, that finding would serve very nicely as an explanation for the meaning of this part of Difficulty 1. What Simonov discovered is that if a practitioner places three fingers on the radial pulse proximal to the styloid process on both the left and right arms simultaneously, then by alternately pressing and releasing the pressure of one's fingers, it is evident that the pulses on the two sides show opposite directionality (i.e., towards the surface or floating vs. towards the interior or sinking), and that this directionality reverses every 14.4 minutes. Thus the movement of the pulse on a given arm cycles, outwards or inwards, every 28.8 minutes, which Simonov calls a period, exactly corresponding to the statements in the *Nan Jing*. On a given arm the 28.8 minute period is obviously divided into two halves, moving outwards for 14.4 minutes and then inwards for 14.4 minutes, or vice-versa. Simonov uses the term "cut" (kè 刻) for this 14.4 minute segment.[13] Simonov additionally found that these 28.8 minute periods are synchronized, as reflected in the

13 刻 kè originally meant a quarter, and as we shall see, the model Simonov proposes comprises two cuts of a yang period followed by two cuts of a yin period (or vice-versa), making a full yin yang cycle of four quarters (one Chinese hour) in the shape of a sine wave. First the polarity rises for 14.4 minutes, then falls back to baseline for 14.4 minutes, then falls below neutral (switches polarity) for 14.4 minutes, then rises back to baseline for 14.4 minutes, ready to start the cycle over again. Thus a cycle of four quarters makes one hour (57.6 minutes). In the ancient Chinese system there were 25 hours each day, which works out to exactly 1440 minutes, the same duration as our 24 hour

radial arteries of the left and right arms, beginning simultaneously in all people examined in the same location, or indeed any location sharing the same solar noon time, implying that these periods, and the movements they reflect, are environmentally induced by the interaction of the Sun and Earth (which determine our day/night phenomenon) on the radial pulse.

Since each period is composed of two cuts, it would be strongly confirmative of this interpretation if there were a signal in the pulse that coincided with the 28.8 minute period directly, rather than with the 14.4 minute cuts. Simonov once again described a location for such a signal, which he interprets as the original meaning of cùn kǒu.[14] He teaches that the pulse at the acupuncture point LU 9 can be found to be more superficial on either the left or right wrist (corresponding to yang and yin respectively), for exactly 28.8 minutes defining yang and yin periods, and that each of these yang or yin periods starts at the same time as the first cut determined by the previous pulse finding. Thus

---

day of 60 minutes each. Since 25 is an odd number, each half-day starts with a different yin yang period, a phenomenon that would not be apparent using a 24 hour clock. See yabla for the definition of 刻 kè: https://chinese.yabla.com/chinese-english-pinyin-dictionary.php?define=刻.

14 Wieger (1965, p.180, L.72A) gives one primitive form of the character kǒu 口, showing a line dividing into two branches, with a connection on top. Simonov interprets this as the image of the radial artery at the wrist dividing into two branches, one of which forms an anastomosis across the palm with the ulnar artery. An alternating change in the direction of flow in this anastomosis is what Simonov asserts as being the mechanism responsible for the 28.8 minute periodic shift in superficiality and strength of the radial pulse between left (yang) and right (yin) wrists at LU 9, reported by Simonov as reflecting the yang and yin periods. It is possible that cùn kǒu, like other technical terms in Chinese medical theory, had different meanings at different historical times, and in different contexts. I have already given the example of rén yíng being used in several classical texts, with entirely different connotations from each other. The presence of this ambiguity is not evidence that one interpretation of a term is correct and the other is incorrect. They may both be correct when used in the appropriate context.

yang and yin periods alternate in each person every 28.8 minutes (first rising and then falling for 14.4 minutes each), but curiously, when males exhibit a yang period (more superficial LU 9 pulse on the left), females exhibit a yin period (more superficial LU 9 pulse on the right). I have found that this pulse phenomenon, as explained by Simonov, is rather more difficult to perceive than the directionality of the róng and wèi cuts. However, in my experience, the alternation of superficiality from left to right sides every 28.8 minutes does seem to be more easily detected slightly more proximally than Simonov teaches, that is, in the traditional cùn position, conventionally found with the radial edge of the index finger abutting the scaphoid bone (whereas Simonov locates the cùn position more proximally, centered over the styloid process).

The discovery of these 28.8 minute periods allows one (Simonov again) to formulate a hypothesis about another, perhaps even more controversial, statement in Difficulty 1:

> "(In a) human, (for) one exhalation the pulsation travels three cùn, (for) one inhalation the pulsation travels three cùn, (an) exhalation (and an) inhalation make (one) breath, (and the) pulsation travels six cùn. Man makes during every one day and one night 13,500 breaths, (and) pulsation travels fifty times."[15]

This passage has been more or less universally interpreted as referring to pulmonary exhalation and inhalation (for obvious reasons), but there are problems with such an interpretation. 13,500 breaths per 24 hours comes out to 9.375 breaths per minute; however, if one consults any of numerous references on the normal range for respiratory rate, that will be found to generally amount to 16–20 breaths per minute, so the *Nan Jing* rate is about half the

15 The text excerpt reads: 人一呼 脈 行 三 寸 一 吸 脈 行 三 寸 呼 吸 定 息 脈 行 六寸. 人一日一 夜 凡 一 萬 三 千 五 百 息 脈 行五十度. The English is my paraphrasing of Simonov's translation.

rate commonly encountered today.[16] If the ancient Chinese were so accurate with their water clock measurements, enabling them to specify the timing of the yin and yang pulse periods to tenths of a minute, how could they be so far off in measuring the respiratory rate of a normal adult? As Simonov has pointed out, the *Nan Jing* commentary on breath is better interpreted as discussing the movement of qì 氣 and mài 脈 (pulsation) through the meridians, so when it mentions breath, it would be reasonable to consider that it might be referring to the qì (literally breath) of the mài, rather than to the functioning of the Lungs. In this explanation, a "pulse breath" rather than a "pulmonary breath" is what occurs 9.375 times per minute, each pulse breath lasting about 6.4 seconds. I do not think Simonov has reported a pulse finding that can be observed every 6.4 seconds, but he does use this duration for implementing certain needle techniques that I have found to be effective in correcting both imbalances in the pulses and symptoms reported by my patients. My reason for introducing these latter remarks is merely to indicate that the ancient Chinese may have been extremely accurate in their observation of pulse breaths, as opposed to the conventional conclusion that they were poor observers of the respiratory rhythm.

Finally, I'd like to describe one more pulse examination that I find brings a sense of coherency to Simonov's teachings. *Nan Jing* chapter 3 discusses two terms that I have not seen incorporated in the acupuncture practices of any of my other teachers. I'm referring to yin victory (陰乘 yīn chéng) and yang victory (陽乘 yáng chéng). The text describes pulses that either overflow their boundaries, or fail to reach them; however, it neither gives concrete directions for determining the presence of these pulses, nor interprets their significance in the context of following the presentations in the first two chapters of the *Nan Jing* (not to

16 See Medscape: http://emedicine.medscape.com/article/2172054-overview.

mention a lack of guidance in how to employ the recognition of these pulse findings in formulating acupuncture treatments). Simonov discovered that by placing four fingers on the radial artery proximal to the styloid, and then pulling the artery first proximally and then distally, the practitioner will experience one direction as manifesting pulses on more fingers than the opposite direction. If the pulse is felt by more fingers when pulling the artery towards the elbow, that indicates yang victory. If the pulse is felt by more fingers when pulling the artery towards the wrist, that indicates yin victory. The text's explanation is that yang victory means the yang is invading the territory that normally is associated with yin (towards the elbow), while yin victory means the yin is invading the territory that normally is associated with yang (towards the wrist crease). Experientially, what Simonov found (and my experience corroborates), is that both yang victory and yin victory pulse patterns last for 12 hours each, alternating at solar noon. In males, yang victory starts its 12 hour cycle at solar noon, which is then followed by a 12 hour phase of yin victory. In females it is the opposite: solar noon initiates 12 hours of yin victory, followed by 12 hours of yang victory.[17]

All this information would be merely technical trivia without the key to understanding its implications, again discovered (or rediscovered) by Simonov: during yang victory, the human organism is disposed to receive cosmic yang qì if acupuncture needles are placed in appropriately receptive places (acupuncture points), while during yin victory it is cosmic yin qì that can be similarly absorbed. This finding leads to powerful methods of acupuncture treatment, but can be rather confusing at first. The absorbed qì will influence the wèi qì with shallow insertion,

17 To be closer to the traditional viewpoint, the 12 hour cycles start at solar midnight, with yin victory in males and yang victory in females. In practical terms this is equivalent to my presentation above, which I think is an easier presentation to follow.

but will influence the róng qì with deep insertion, so care must be taken to correctly determine the state of the meridian to be needled by attending to whether it is either a yin or a yang meridian, and whether the pulse shows excess or deficiency of the róng qì that normally pertains to that meridian. Although my description of these "victory" states may not provide enough information to begin using this information in clinical practice, the coherent explanation it provides for the understanding of nature's rhythms, as expressed in the opening chapters of the *Nan Jing*, will hopefully encourage more practitioners to study Simonov's work in depth.

The overall picture that I see in this interpretation of the beginning chapters of the *Nan Jing* is that of cycles within cycles. The biggest cycle is that of the 24 hour alternation of day and night. This cycle is composed of two halves (yin victory and yang victory) that represent the cosmic impact on humans of yin and yang qi, and which can be verified by the four-finger pulse exam. Each half-day is composed of 25 alternating periods of yin or yang nature, representing times when the qi is predominantly in either the yin or yang meridians, and which can be verified by a comparison of the pulse at (or near) the LU 9 acupuncture point between left and right wrists. These yin or yang periods last 28.8 minutes each, and have two parts called cuts of 14.4 minutes each. For example, in a yang period, the yang is always greater than the yin, but during the first cut it is increasing, while during the second cut it is decreasing back towards equality with the yin. These cuts can also be verified by pressing and lifting one's fingers on both left and right radial pulses, proximal to the styloid. There is additionally a 6.4 second pulse breath alluded to in these first few chapters, which has clinical importance for acupuncture practice, but for which there is no palpatory method of verification discovered yet, to my knowledge.

Now let us jump to chapter 50 of the *Nan Jing*, which I see as laying the theoretical groundwork for understanding the difference between constitutional and conditional aspects of diagnosis in Oriental medicine. Although constitutional types were presented in *Ling Shu* chapters 64 and 72, in terms of yin-yang and Five Element theories, it is not clear whether these types were thought of as inborn or acquired. In addition, there were no practical guidelines given for determining the constitutional type, nor for adopting anything more than the most general rules for treating people of different types.[18] In the twentieth century, this distinction between constitution (inborn) and condition (acquired) was made the explicit basis for two systematized approaches to acupuncture: the Five Element style codified by Worsley in England, and the KCA style developed by Kuon in Korea. Both of these approaches to acupuncture practice can be viewed as developments based on what I consider the "radical" model introduced in *Nan Jing* 50. The reason I use the word "radical" is that, for the first time, a classical text focused on the systematic relationship between the various Organ systems as being of primary concern, rather than simply localizing a symptom/sign complex to one of them. In other words, any Organ system (or meridian) can affect any other Organ system (or meridian), and as a result, any specific illness or symptom/sign complex could have its root anywhere among the zàng fŭ. This is what I call a "constellational" interpretation of physiology, pathology, diagnosis and treatment formulation.

18 The constitutional types are described in the *Ling Shu* in terms of physical characteristics, behavioral characteristics, and susceptibility to disease, using both yin yang and wu xing theories. Some contemporary styles of Oriental medicine, such as Sa Sang Constitutional Medicine, emphasize physical body type (tǐ zhì 體質) in constitutional diagnosis, while others use either pulse diagnosis (KCA) or color, sound of voice, odor, and emotion (Worsley's Five Element style of acupuncture) as primary discriminators in constitutional diagnosis.

Here is what chapter 50 says:[19]

> "Among the illnesses are the deficiency (xū) evil, the excess (shí) evil, the usurper (zéi) evil, the declining (wēi) evil, and the principal (zhèng) evil. How can they be distinguished? It is like this: Those coming from behind represent a deficiency evil; those coming from ahead represent an excess evil; those coming from what cannot be overcome represent a usurper evil; those coming from what can be overcome represent a declining evil; if affected from within itself, that represents a principal evil."[20]

An example is given in chapter 50 that uses Heart disease originating from various causes as an illustration. The text cites exogenous evils (wind, immoderate eating, cold, damp, and heat) as illustrative causes, but it should always be kept in mind that the fundamental principle of resonance (gǎn yìng) implies that one could equally well cite the Liver, Spleen, Kidney, Lung, or Heart as causes of the manifested Heart disease. In fact, most of the commentaries on this chapter in Unschuld's translation cite these Organ relationships explicitly. What does this broader, resonance-inspired interpretation imply? To me it is obviously saying that Heart disease can come from any Organ, and by extension, so can any illness, be it diabetes, asthma, hepatitis, and more. This underlying cause is, in other words, the root cause of the illness, and the idea of constitutional diagnosis

---

19 五十難曰: 病有虛邪, 有實邪, 有賊邪, 有微邪, 有正邪, 何以別之? 然: 從後來者為虛邪, 從前來者為實邪, 從所不勝來者為賊邪, 從所勝來者為微邪, 自病者為正邪.

20 The author's translation. There are many choices of names for these five evils, but I have picked the ones that I think best reflect the spirit of this chapter, which is to flesh out the concepts of xiāng shēng and xiāng kè in a clinical context. The idea of tonification and sedation points (and the "mother–son law") is a natural corollary of this passage, as is the subsequently developed Korean four-needle technique, which additionally uses the grandparent to oppose its grandchild.

is specifically to identify the root causes of illness regardless of its specific manifestation.

Another way of saying this is that each of us has a unique original nature. Anything that takes us away from our original nature is moving us toward illness, while anything that brings us back to our original nature is moving us toward health. I have found in my practice that one of the most reliable indicators of healing is not whether a particular symptom is diminished or even goes away, but rather when the patient spontaneously exclaims, "Oh! I feel like myself again." Remember that, in a way, the same idea was expressed in the *Nei Jing* regarding the significance of pulse changes over symptom changes in prognostication: if the pulse becomes more normal, even if the symptom doesn't change, the prognosis is favorable; but if the pulse doesn't improve, even if the symptom does, the prognosis is unfavorable.

Chapter 50 can thus be seen as the inspiration for Worsley's Five Element style focus on what he called the Causative Factor (CF). The CF is the source of the various "evils" that can result in imbalances in any of the Elements or Organ systems in the body, and therefore treatment to restore the CF to proper functioning (its original nature) is the route to healing. Of course, such a statement is a huge simplification of a complex style of acupuncture, but recognizing this root schema in chapter 50 is responsible for the vast difference in approach between Five Element style acupuncture and TCM acupuncture. I remember being quite skeptical when Worsley repeatedly claimed that any symptom can come from any Organ or Element, but my clinical experience supports his contention.

KCA, developed by Kuon Dowon, adopts essentially the same idea (anything can come from anything), but develops it in a different manner so as to articulate the relationship between the underlying constitution and the presenting condition (symptom or illness). I will again use the word "constellational" to describe its conceptualization. Let us take Excess Liver as the constitutional diagnosis. In KCA, all inflammatory disorders of the Fǔ Organs (including gastritis, colitis, sinusitis, endometritis, etc.) in an individual of Liver Excess type are treated as problems of Liver "usurping" the Spleen, to use the terminology of chapter 50. To give another example, if the constitution is diagnosed as Heart Excess, then these same Fǔ Organ problems would be treated as Heart usurping the Lung.[21] KCA is much more complex, with different constellational treatments for inflammation of the Zang Organs, neuro-psychological problems, infections, acute and chronic pains, and simple trauma. By constellational, I mean that the Kidney can be the conditional cause for degenerative illnesses in one person (Liver Excess constitution), nephrosis in another (Kidney Deficiency constitution), pancreatitis in a third (Heart Excess constitution), cystitis in a fourth (Spleen Deficiency constitution), and cervical disc disease in a fifth (Large Intestine Deficiency constitution). From this brief description, the reader can see that KCA incorporated aspects of Chinese medicine, Korean (Sa Sang) medicine, and even Western medicine.

Notwithstanding this heterogeneous approach, the central focus of KCA is on determining the constitution (original nature), and this is essentially accomplished via a unique style of pulse diagnosis, identifying a signature in the pulse that never changes throughout the life of each individual. Finally, I should mention that Kuon cited the *Nan Jing* as an inspiration in developing KCA, and I see this style of practice as a good example of using the empirical experience of touch (pulse diagnosis) as the foundation of an Eastern scientific approach to acupuncture as a vehicle for healthcare.

---

21 I am using the formulation of Constitutional Acupuncture I proposed in *The Compleat Acupuncturist* (Eckman 2014). It represents a development based on Kuon's original methodology, but does not strictly follow any of the subsequent iterations of his methods, which he now calls Eight Constitutions Medicine.

Chapter 7

Mài Jīng 脈經

THE PULSE CLASSIC

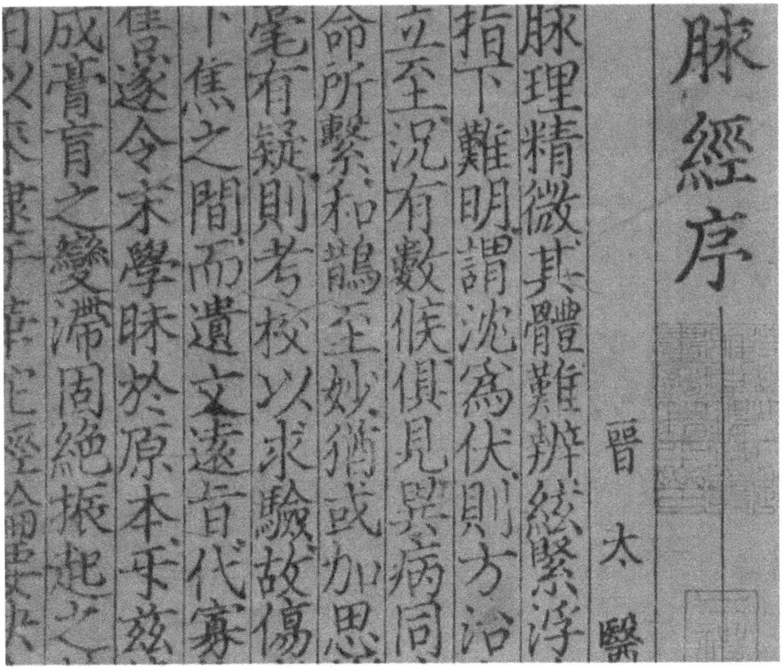
脉經序

晉太醫

脉理精微其體難辨絃緊浮
指下難明謂沈爲伏則方治
立至況有數候俱見異病同
命所繫和鵲至妙猶或加思
毫有疑則考校以求驗故傷
下焦之間而遺文遠旨代寡
售遂令末學昧於原本斥茲
成膏肓之變滯固絕振起之

Figure 7.1 Yuan dynasty copy of *Mai Jing*[1]
Source: World Digital Library

1 This Yuan dynasty edition, based on the earlier edition by Lin Yi, was printed by Guangqin Shutang in Jianyang, Fujian, in 1330, and is considered the earliest extant printed copy. 脉 is an alternate form of mài 脈.

The *Mai Jing* (a text composed of 10 Books with their own Chapters) was written by Wang Shuhe c.280 CE, making it a later work than the *Nan Jing*, from which it borrowed whole chapters. An English translation by Yang Shouzhong was first published in 1997 (Yang 1997). In his Foreword, the translator acknowledged that there were several versions of the Chinese text, from which he selected the statements and interpretations that made the most sense (to him), and he pointed out that ancient Chinese was so terse and cryptic that multiple interpretations of even basic terms are in fact possible. Chapters 3 and 4 of Book 1 of the *Mai Jing* are almost identical in wording and content to chapters 1 through 3 of the *Nan Jing*, but allow enough latitude to support the interpretation I have proposed for the locations of cùn kǒu and the three places known as cùn, guān, and chǐ, as I will try to demonstrate. Unfortunately I only have a partial copy of the Chinese text, so my interpretation is speculative at best.

Mai Jing Book 1, chapter 3 states:

> "Where pulse may be examined is a master place divided in three sections. From the fish margin (wrist crease) to the high bone (styloid), retreat back one cùn. In front is a place named cùn kǒu."[2]

What is the significance of mentioning the fish margin in relation to the master place, and then retreating back one cùn from the styloid? The only way I can make sense of this passage is to assume that it is discussing the region from the wrist crease to one cùn proximal to the styloid as the chǐ cùn region, where practitioners feel the three sections named cùn, guān, and chǐ. This territory occupies approximately two inches, which by proportional measurement is more or less the same as the width of the three examining fingers. The intention here appears to me to use *back*

2 脉候所主第三从魚際至高骨却行一寸其中名曰寸口.

to mean *proximal* and *front* to mean *distal*. Starting from the wrist crease, one cùn back would place the location at the styloid, and retreating back one cùn more would place the location at the proximal end of the chǐ cùn region. In front of (distal to) this location would thus indicate the entire region chǐ cùn, which is then asserted to be the location of cùn kǒu. This passage would appear to disagree with Simonov's identification of the location of cùn kǒu as the LU 9 acupuncture point on the wrist crease, but rather support the interpretation of cùn kǒu as the whole region for pulse examination encompassing cùn, guān, and chǐ.[3]

When we come to Book 10, the description of cùn kǒu appears to corroborate my interpretation of its meaning and location. The English translation of this passage in Book 10 reads:

> "The cùn opening (cùn kǒu) is the place where yin and yang meet. (The cùn opening) is divided into five portions. The distal and the proximal (positions), the left and right (sides), each rules something. Based on the upper (i.e., the cùn), the lower (i.e., the chǐ), and the middle (i.e., the guān), there is a division of nine portions."[4]

While the specific meaning of the five portions and the nine portions is open to question, there appears to be no way to

---

3 Simonov disagrees on the location of the cùn position. He places cùn directly at the crest of the styloid, although I can't see how the text implies this interpretation. *Mai Jing* Book 1 chapter 4 states, "from guān to the fish margin is the sphere of cùn." Since cùn has been assigned a length of 0.9 inches, this would appear to refer to the distance from the fish margin to the styloid. Simonov's interpretation is that in the initial chapters of both texts (*Nan Jing* and *Mai Jing*), cùn kǒu is differentiated from cùn, guān, and chǐ, and rather than serving as a place to diagnose the Organs or meridians, is rather a place (LU 9) that serves to control the alternate periods of yin and yang of 28.8 minutes each.

4 寸口之中陰陽交會中有五部．前後左右各有所主上下中央分為九道．See Figure 7.2 for an illustration from Book 10 of the nine portions.

interpret this description of cùn kǒu as referring to the pulse at the wrist crease location (LU 9). Rather, cùn kǒu in this case seems to clearly refer to the composite locations of cùn, guān, and chǐ. We are left needing to recognize that cùn kǒu might have multiple meanings, even within the same text, and that how we interpret its meaning must be dependent on the context.

The text above initially mentions five portions (部 bù), with the subsequent sentence referring to distal, proximal, left, and right. This brings to mind the arrangement of the Five Elements (wǔxíng) with top, bottom, left, right, and center (implied), which correspond to Fire, Water, Wood, Metal, and Earth respectively. Will Morris has published his research on using these five directions (where the pulse is clearest or most congested at any of the six positions) to identify Elemental imbalances, using what he has called the "compass method."[5] The sentence after the five portions mentions nine portions (分 fēn) consisting of upper, lower, and middle, illustrated in Figure 7.2. These three positions correlate with cùn, chǐ, and guān respectively, and each of them has a center, radial, and ulnar location, leading to nine portions. The English editor notes that these nine portions are not the same as the "nine indicators."[6]

5 www.acupuncturetoday.com/mpacms/at/article.php?id=28028.

6 The "nine indicators" was Unschuld's translation of a term appearing in *Nan Jing* chapter 18 (九候 jiǔ hòu), where it was introduced but not explained. Various commentators have proposed that the nine indicators there refer to the superficial, middle, and deep pulses at cùn, guān, and chǐ. In Book 4, chapter 1 of the *Mai Jing*, the nine indicators are identified as the Heaven, Earth and Man of cùn, guān, and chǐ, and make explicit reference to depth in at least one passage. It is certainly possible that the *Nan Jing* commentators were influenced by these statements in the *Mai Jing*. The "nine portions" thus refer to horizontal positions at cùn, guān, and chǐ, while the "nine indicators" refer to vertical positions at these same three locations.

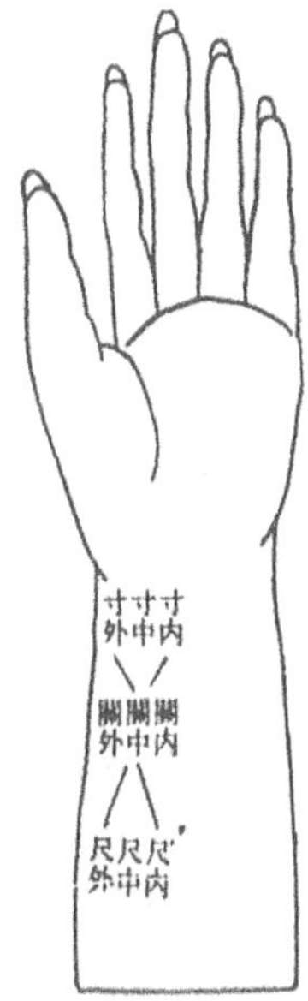

Figure 7.2 The nine portions in Book 10 of *Mai Jing*
Source: Yang 1997

Although the *Mai Jing* did not repeat the terminology of nine portions (jiŭ fēn 九分) in its immediately following descriptions of the locations from radial to middle to ulnar (i.e., left, center, and right, or vice-versa, depending on which wrist is being discussed) at cùn, guān, and chǐ, it did correlate these positions with the beating of the pulses of the principal meridians in this passage from Book 10.[7] This presentation of nine portions is certainly problematic, in that it allocates positions for evaluating the pulses corresponding to only nine of the twelve principal meridians. I imagine every serious student of this text must have immediately asked themselves, "What about the other three principal meridians' pulses?" Moreover, Book 1 chapter 7 and Book 3 had already

7 前如外者, 足太陽也; 中央如外者, 足陽明也; 後如外者, 足少陽也. 中央直前者, 手少陰也; 中央直中者, 手心主也; 中央直後者, 手太陰也. 前如內者, 足厥陰也; 中央如內者, 足太陰也. 後如內者, 足少陰也.

specified the pulse positions at cùn, guān, and chǐ, for the zàng fǔ and their corresponding meridians, and those positions are at variance with the assignments in Book 10. Unfortunately, the *Mai Jing* does not give an explanation of, nor justification for, these different schemata. Book 10 also presents other puzzling issues. Even its title is a mystery: "Hand Diagram of the Thirty-One Positions." What are the thirty-one positions, and how does their description mesh with that of the previous chapters, and of other classical texts? Finally, what is the meaning of the lines in Figure 7.2 connecting the central position at guān with the inner and outer (ulnar and radial) positions at cùn, and chǐ?[8] I believe there are reasonable answers to each of these questions, which I will describe as hypotheses that have proven useful in my clinical practice.

Before presenting my proposed answers to these puzzling questions, I should point out that the history of commentaries on the classical Chinese medical texts is one of multiple interpretations, often directly conflicting with each other, and sometimes even going so far as to call the original text nonsensical.[9] The extant texts are also of questionable accuracy, as there were often omissions, character mistakes by copyists, and personal interpretations (including additions, both acknowledged and unacknowledged) by editors.[10] These commentators were for the most part seasoned practitioners with a great deal of clinical experience, so it is entirely within the tradition for me to question the accuracy of at least one

8 I am indebted to Andrew Prescott for calling my attention to these last two questions.

9 See Unschuld (1986) for a sample of contentious commentaries.

10 The postscript to the version of the *Mai Jing* compiled by He Da-ren in 1217 stated, "...a good edition of this classic has been a rarity. All the versions available abound in mistakes and typographical errors...in the collection of my family, there was a copy of the edition published...in the reign of Shao Sheng (1094–1098). This copy, old of age, was worn out and abraded, and it was impossible that there were not any miswritten characters in it" (Yang 1997, p.363).

part of the passage describing the nine portions. This is an excellent example of how I envision Oriental science in action: not relying on abstract hypotheses, even of revered authorities, as the ultimate way to truth, but rather paying close attention to clinical observations (the map is not the territory).

Some background regarding the material covered in the *Mai Jing* will be helpful in understanding my hypotheses. Its author, Wang Shuhe, relied on texts from the *Nei Jing*, *Nan Jing*, and *Shang Han Lun* (and presumably other lost texts) in compiling the pulse teachings of the *Mai Jing*. The first two of these texts are primarily concerned with acupuncture, and the third is primarily concerned with herbal medicine, and while their theoretical bases share much in common, there are also divergent teachings, so Wang had a difficult task in synthesizing a text reflective of the theories governing both modalities of treatment.

Among the topics discussed in the *Mai Jing* are the following. Book 1, chapter 7 describes the locations of the pulses associated with the twelve zàng fũ (and mentions their associated hand or foot meridians in terms of the six energetic levels [SEL] of yin and yang). These associations (Table 7.1) are then confirmed and expanded upon in the five chapters of Book 3 in terms of their Five Element (wǔxíng) resonances (pulse quality, spiritual faculty, color, tissue nourished, sensory portal, sound, odor, fluid discharge, flavor, season, time of day, and direction). Incidentally, the Back Shu Points and Front Mo Points of all the zàng fũ (except for those of Ming Men and San Jiao) are also specified there for the first time. Book 2, chapter 4, in the interim, describes the pulses of the eight extraordinary vessels (qí jīng bā mài 奇經八脈). The translator of the English edition added a footnote stating, "one should not feel these images (i.e., the extraordinary vessel pulses) in normal cases. If a pulse of an extraordinary vessel is present, some disorder related to that vessel already does exist" (Yang 1997, p.57). Book 4, chapter 1 introduces the nine indicators (jiǔ hòu 九候) as an informative model for interpreting pulses at three depths at each of cùn, guān, and chǐ (depths emblematic of Heaven, Man, and Earth respectively). Finally, Book 10 begins by summarizing the contents of the preceding chapters, but then adds a new (i.e., different) association of pulse location and hand or foot SEL meridian, which it calls the nine portions (jiǔ fēn 九分), shown in Table 7.2.

TABLE 7.1 PULSE LOCATIONS ACCORDING TO *MAI JING* BOOKS 1 AND 3

	Left wrist		*Right wrist*	
Cùn	Heart Small Intestine	Hand Shao Yin Hand Tai Yang	Lung Large Intestine	Hand Tai Yin Hand Yang Ming
Guān	Liver Gall Bladder	Foot Jue Yin Foot Shao Yang	Spleen Stomach	Foot Tai Yin Foot Yang Ming
Chǐ	Kidney Urinary Bladder	Foot Shao Yin Foot Tai Yang	Life Gate/ Kidney Sanjiao/Bladder	? ?

TABLE 7.2 PULSE LOCATIONS ACCORDING TO *MAI JING* BOOK 10

Location	*Meridian*
Outer Cùn	Foot Tai Yang (UB)
Central Cùn	Hand Shao Yin (HE)
Inner Cùn	Foot Jue Yin (LV)
Outer Guān	Foot Yang Ming (ST)
Central Guān	Hand Heart Governor
Inner Guān	Foot Tai Yin (SP)
Outer Chǐ	Foot Shao Yang (GB)
Central Chǐ	Hand Tai Yin (LU)
Inner Chǐ	Foot Shao Yin (KI)

The first question I'll address is the identity of the 31 positions (bù 部) in the title of Book 10. Since there is no discussion of the connecting meridians (luò mài 絡脈), divergent meridians (jīng bié 經別), or tendino-muscular meridians (jīng jiàn 經腱), I think we can eliminate them from consideration. The text describes nine portions (jiǔ fēn 九分) on both left and right, making 18 positions. It also describes five portions (wǔ bù 五部), leaving eight positions. There are exactly eight extraordinary pulses described, bringing the total to 31. Let us keep in mind that the nine portions refer to a yin yang categorization pertaining to the SEL, while the five portions refer to a Five Element categorization. That is the dynamic that Wang needed to synthesize. I pointed out as early as 1983, in *Closing the Circle* (Eckman 1983), that herbal medicine is a yin modality with respect to acupuncture, which is a yang modality, and that yin yang theory (2 is a yin number) is relatively yin with respect to Five Element theory (5 is a yang number), which is relatively yang.[11] Thus Wang was striving to present a synthesis of both cardinal theories and therapeutic modalities of CM, but did not omit their root (on an embryological or pre-heavenly level) in the eight extraordinary meridians that play a crucial role in the development of both the zàng fǔ and the jīng mài, a topic that I will touch on in the Addendum.

When we look at the manifestation of yin and yang in terms of directionality along the radial artery, one aspect is obvious: yin resonates with interior, which in this case is toward the ulnar direction (little finger), while yang resonates with exterior, which in this case is towards the radial direction (thumb). This interpretation agrees perfectly with six of the nine positions

11 The radical for both yin and yang depicts a hill (fǔ 阜), which is a structure, while the character for element or phase (xíng 行), which is also a radical, refers specifically to an activity, that is, movement. See Wieger (1965) Lesson 86A for 阜, and Lesson 63C for 行.

shown in Table 7.2. A problem arises, however, when we try to understand the associations given for the three remaining positions described as central. Central does not resonate with yin or yang in this case (being the balance point between them), but all three of these positions are correlated with hand yin meridians (Heart, Heart Governor, and Lung), while the three hand yang meridians (Small Intestine, Sanjiao, and Large Intestine) are omitted from the analysis. Is there any possible way of resolving this conundrum?

In *The Compleat Acupuncturist* (Eckman 2014) I presented a schema of the associations relating to the six energetic levels (SEL), which I've classified as radial or ulnar deviations, as specified in the *Mai Jing* in its presentation of the nine portions (jiǔ fēn 九分). In the years of additional clinical observation since my proposed schema was written, I have repeatedly confirmed my hypothesis, which I now repeat here (positions 1, 2, and 3 corresponding to cùn, guān, and chǐ respectively), as shown in Table 7.3 and Figure 7.3.

TABLE 7.3 THE SEL DEVIATIONS

Deviation	*Meridian*
Radial Cùn	Tai Yang (UB and SI)
Radial Guān	Yang Ming (ST and LI)
Radial Chǐ	Shao Yang (GB and TH)
Ulnar Cùn	Jue Yin (LV and PE)
Ulnar Guān	Tai Yin (SP and LU)
Ulnar Chǐ	Shao Yin (KI and HE)

The yin and yang SEL assignments given by the *Mai Jing* for the foot meridians are correct, and what I have found is that they are equally applicable to the hand meridians as well. Additionally, there is no particular association with the central position between radial and ulnar directions, as the center has no association with yin or yang in this context. This finding is analogous to that of the *Nei Jing*'s presentation of RYCK diagnostic patterns, where the hand and foot branches of the same SEL meridian show identical proportionality; it is only the pulse quality that changes, depending on whether a foot or hand branch is imbalanced.

In the case of radial or ulnar deviation of the radial artery, once again the SEL indicated is the same for hand and foot branches, but I have not as yet identified a difference in pulse quality for differentiating hand vs. foot branch. My hypothesis was developed as part of the search for pulse indicators of an individual's constitutional typology, and I should point out that the *Mai Jing* does not indicate which aspect of a meridian's nature is related to the presence of radial or ulnar deviations. It could be a constitutional indicator (as I have found it to be), or it could reflect some other state, such as an abnormality of the wèi qì in the corresponding tendino-muscular meridian (a conditional, rather than constitutional, state) as I was taught by Joseph Adams, and attributed by him to Will Morris.

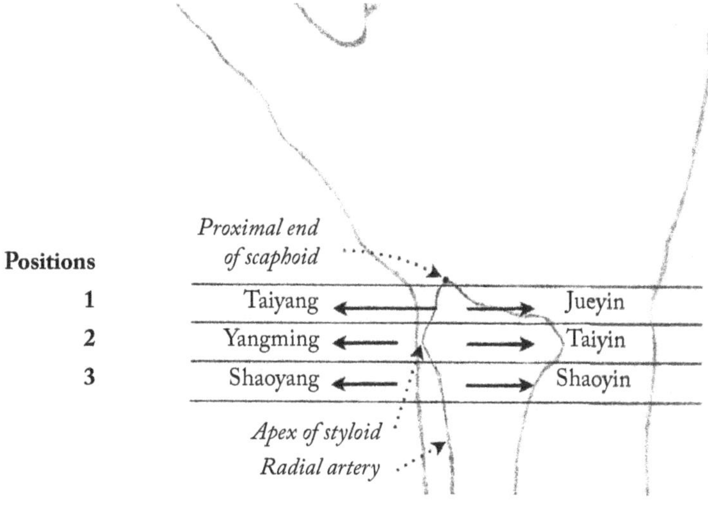

Figure 7.3 SEL radial and ulnar deviations
Source: Neal White and Peter Eckman

These deviations in the architecture of the radial artery can be thought of as a standing wave form, and I have found the identical waveform to be present when the examiner moves their fingers proximally one "wavelength" to what I call positions 4, 5, and 6. This repeated waveform can be a useful check on whether the examiner's fingers are in the correct position or not, and also as a way to confirm the SEL constitutional diagnosis. There is one exception to this repeated waveform in my experience, and that is when there is an activation of any of the extraordinary vessels, a topic I will address presently. First it is necessary to describe the criteria I use for correct finger placement at positions 1, 2, and 3 (cùn, guān, and chǐ).

In my *JCM* article (Eckman 2015), I pointed out that precise finger position in evaluating cùn, guān, and chǐ is crucial for obtaining accurate readings, and this applies equally whether palpating for depth of the pulse or deviation of the pulse at any of these three locations. In summary, the guān position is directly over the crest of the styloid process, but the cùn and chǐ positions need to be adjusted to the patient's anatomy relative to that of the examiner.[12] The possible variations are illustrated in Figures 7.4, 7.5, and 7.6.

12 Since publication of this article, I have discovered that there is a more accurate method for determining the gap or overlap of the examiner's fingers, one which depends on the relative width of the examiner's fingers compared to the width of the patient's fingers, consistent with the traditional notion of proportionality (i.e., the "body inch" or "cùn"). If the examiner's fingers are narrower than the patient's (Figure 7.5), then the examiner needs to spread their fingers proportionately. If the examiner's fingers are wider than the patient's (Figure 7.6), then the examiner needs to overlap their fingers proportionately. I should add that the finger positions I am describing here are what I call the "yang pulse positions." There is also a more proximal location of cùn, guān, and chǐ, determined by having the examiner's index and middle fingers lie on either side of the crest of the styloid, which I call the "yin pulse positions." The "yin pulse positions," however, are not used in SEL determination by radial or ulnar deviation. As noted, these deviations reflect meridian energetics (SEL), and one

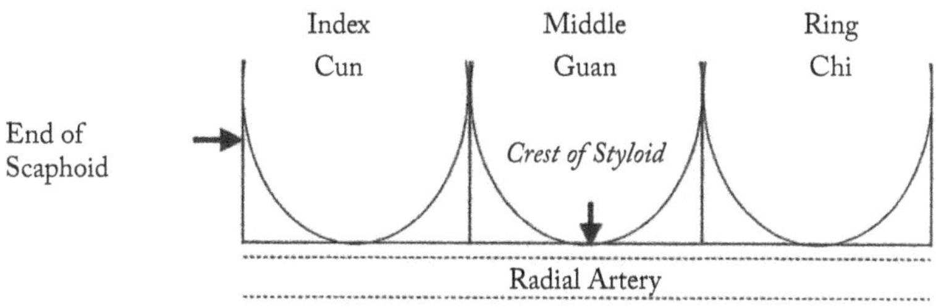

Figure 7.4 Typical (Yang) finger positions for patient of equal finger width as the examiner[13]
Source: Peter Eckman

It is evident in Figures 7.5 and 7.6 that sometimes there will be a gap between the examiner's fingers, while at other times it will be necessary for the examiner to overlap (or underlap) their fingers. With the fingers thus correctly positioned, there should be one finger whose pulse is out of line (parallel to the radial artery) with the other two, deviating either radially or ulnarly, as shown in Figure 7.3, and this deviated pulse indicates which one of the six levels of yin and yang is constitutionally the most vulnerable.

might reasonably classify the meridians as being more yang than the Organs to which they pertain (which are relatively more yin), thus providing a possible rationale for using the "yang pulse positions" to evaluate the lateral deviations correlated with the SEL. The interpretation of the "yang pulse positions" and the "yin pulse positions" will be addressed further in the Addendum.

13 In Figures 7.3, 7.4, 7.5, 7.6, and 7.7 the essential landmark is the crest of the styloid process, which marks the center of the guān position. The relationship with the proximal edge of the scaphoid may not be exactly as depicted. In contrast to the recommendations of the Shen–Hammer teachings to be found in Hammer's publications (Hammer 2001; Hammer and Bilton 2012), I rely only on the styloid process as a landmark and not at all on the scaphoid bone, making adjustments in my index and ring fingers based on the relative width of the patient's fingers to my own.

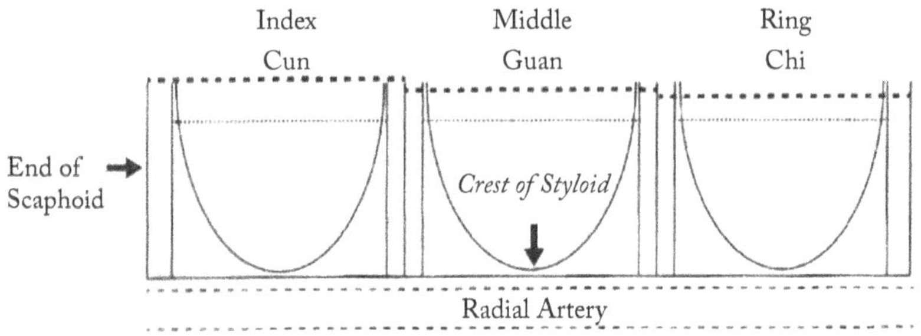

Figure 7.5 Examiner has narrower fingers
Source: Peter Eckman

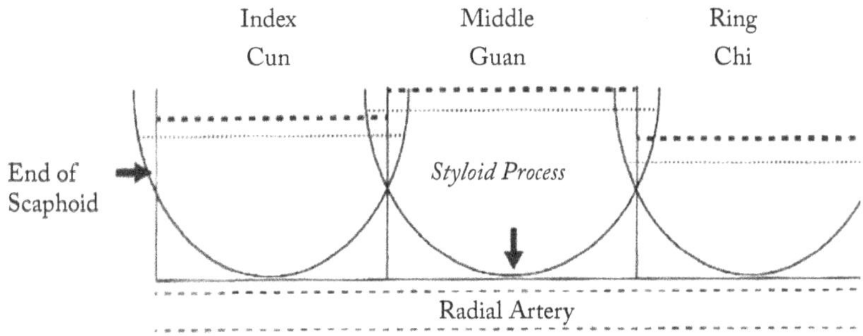

Figure 7.6 Examiner has wider fingers
Source: Peter Eckman

The lines in Figure 7.2, connecting the middle of the guān position with the radial and ulnar (outer and inner) sides of the cùn and chǐ position, appear to me to once again be referencing the Earth-centered arrangement of the Five Elements (wǔxíng). One interpretation of the central, and special, role played by the Earth Element, is that it acts as the transition between each of the other Elements. This format is reflected in the assignment of the seasonal correspondences to the Elements. Some text passages state that the last part of each season is correlated (resonates) with the Earth Element, so that from Wood to Fire, for example, (Spring to Summer) first transits through Earth. Thus, the central spot at guān is Earth. The other four Elements (non-central) must connect through this center in order to influence each other. That, at least, is my interpretation of the lines in Figure 7.2.

So far, I have not presented the pulse patterns of the eight extraordinary vessels as detailed in the *Mai Jing* Books 4 and 10 (Figure 7.7). The text presents several variants of the extraordinary vessel pulses, from which I have selected the following descriptions:

> "A pulse floating in the chǐ to the cùn, (beating) straight up and down, is a governing vessel pulse… If the pulse is firm from the chǐ to the cùn, (beating) straight up and down, this is a pulse of the penetrating vessel… If the pulse arrives tight, fine, replete and long (from the chǐ) to the guān, this is a pulse of the conception vessel."[14]

> "Striking (forcefully) at both the left and right (i.e., outer and inner) side of the distal position is the yang motility (vessel pulse). Striking (forcefully) at both the left and right (i.e., outer and inner) side of the middle position is the girdling (dai) vessel pulse. Striking (forcefully) at both the left and right (i.e., outer and inner) side of the proximal position is the yin motility pulse. From the (foot) shao yang to the (foot) jue yin beats the yin linking (vessel). From the (foot) shao yin to the (foot) tai yang beats the yang linking (vessel)."[15]

14 These descriptions are selected from several described in Book 4. Following Morris's teachings (apparently based on later descriptions by Li Shizhen—see www.acupuncturetoday.com/mpacms/at/article.php?id=27903), I have interpreted these three pulses' patterns as follows: if all three positions are equally superficial, it indicates the governing vessel; if all three are felt equally at the moderate level, it indicates the conception vessel; and if all three are felt equally at the deep level, it indicates the penetrating vessel.

15 These descriptions of the remaining five extraordinary vessel pulses are from Book 10.

These extraordinary vessel pulses, when present, can be detected at cùn, guān, and chǐ. If extraordinary vessel pulses are present, then the SEL pattern of deviation at cùn, guān, and chǐ will no longer be apparent, but interestingly, they will still be detectable at positions 4, 5, and 6, which is one reason why I have introduced these more proximal sites for pulse examination (Figure 7.7). In my experience, after the extraordinary vessels are treated successfully, the SEL pulses can once again be found at positions 1, 2, and 3.

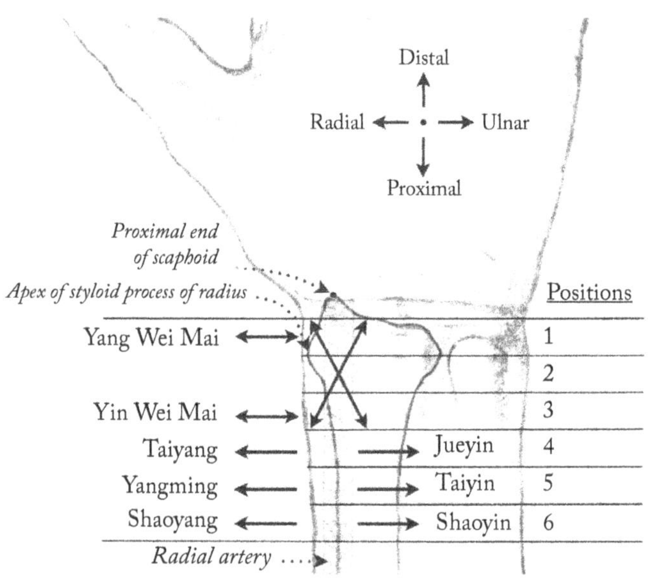

Figure 7.7 SEL deviations and eight extra pulses
Source: Peter Eckman

In summary, I have proposed explanations for three types of pulse patterns described in the *Mai Jing*. The radial (yang) or ulnar (yin) deviations of the pulse positions at cùn, guān, or chǐ on the horizontal plane described in Book 10 indicate which of the SEL are constitutionally vulnerable, and thus appear to be at the "root" of an individual's energetic pathology. Also on the horizontal plane, but on the smaller scale of an individual pulse position, the five directions (proximal, distal, radial, ulnar, and central) of the pulse appear to indicate which of the Five Elements are out of coordination with the "root," thus pointing to the current "branch" or conditional energetic pathology. Finally, if no radial or ulnar deviation is detected at the standard pulse positions (cùn, guān, and chǐ, then an extraordinary vessel imbalance is probably in need of treatment, and can be identified by the pulse pattern it produces.

This discussion of the *Mai Jing* by no means covers the vast amount of information contained in that classic text. However, in the *Mai Jing*, many teachings, including the vertical correlations of pulse depth with the Five Elements and their associated Organs (Book 1, chapter 6), are reprised from the *Nan Jing*, and additionally support the hypotheses I have proposed for understanding Book 10. The order of the SEL deviations in Book 10 might seem mysterious at first, but it has a very simple logic to it. If one looks again at Figure 7.2, the deviations that are diagonally opposite each other can be seen to indicate coupled meridians. Thus Tai Yang is opposite Shao Yin, Yang Ming is opposite Tai Yin, and Shao Yang is opposite Jue Yin. This formation suggests several of the treatment options used in Master Dong (董) style acupuncture that were popularized by the late Richard Tan.

Addendum

Pinning the Tail on the Donkey

I have tried to accomplish two goals in writing this treatise. The first is to provide an introduction to some of the possibly misunderstood passages in the classical texts in the Chinese medical tradition, along with my speculations as to their meaning, based on more than 40 years of clinical practice as an acupuncturist. The second is to try to promote an understanding of Eastern medicine as being based on a scientific approach, albeit a different aspect of science than is characteristic of Western medicine. To that end, I would like to communicate some corrections to my previous publication, *The Compleat Acupuncturist*, which I had described at the time as a work in progress (as is this one, not to put too fine a point on it). Correcting imperfections in theory and practice are at the heart of any scientific endeavor, so this "mea culpa" is meant to illustrate what possibilities are opened up by viewing Eastern medicine as scientific in nature. In no way am I insinuating that any of my writings belongs in the pantheon of classical Chinese medical texts. Familiarity with my previous work would be a distinct advantage in contemplating this Addendum, but is not strictly necessary, as some of my remarks are meant to tie together the material in the different chapters of this treatise, while at the same time maintaining congruity with what I've previously written.

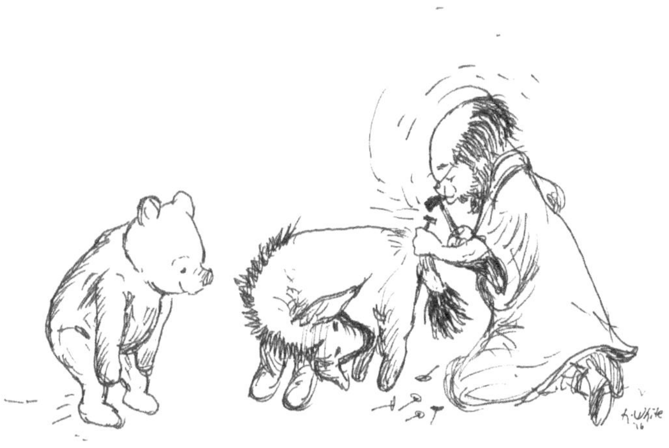

Figure A.1 Pinning the tail on the donkey[1]
Source: Neal White

1 The image parodies E.H Shepherd's original *Winnie the Pooh* illustration. "Eeyore is a favorite amongst most admirers of *Winnie the Pooh* characters and he is an unbelievably loveable donkey who is dismally gloomy for almost eternity. But that's not Eeyore's perception of himself, according to him; he doesn't expect too much of himself and therefore remains quiet for most of the time. That in no ways means he isn't an intelligent animal, he is actually quite knowledgeable yet he confines his knowledge to himself. Eeyore's biggest problem is when his tail falls off and that happens frequently (he has lost it many times). And this is where his friends help him the most and amongst all friends Christopher Robin is the one who mostly undertakes the job of fixing Eeyore's tail. Christopher uses a drawing pin to reattach the tail. It is well known that Eeyore has a depressive nature and he is always gloomy, but he is also a compassionate animal. This is shown when Eeyore is able to grow a plant which Rabbit, a much respected gardener is unable to grow. Eeyore achieves this by giving the plant some of his love." Quoted from www.just-pooh.com/eeyore.html. The reader might like to ponder Eeyore's relationship to Daoist philosophy, especially to the hypothesis that love is the vehicle of total resonance. I am not the first to see a reflection of Daoism in A.A. Milne's beloved text. Benjamin Hoff's *The Tao of Pooh* and *The Te of Piglet* got there before I did, but only saw Eeyore as fretful. My own take is that we all have a bit of enlightenment interwoven in our makeup, the recognition of which is the first step in our individual spiritual development.

Let me begin by re-establishing the basic distinction between a person's constitution and their condition. Although many approaches to medical practice are simply focused on alleviating the presenting condition (which is not in itself a bad idea), it is my conviction that the ultimate goal of any medical intervention should be to help return each person to their original nature, which I have been calling their constitution.[2] Unless attention is paid to discovering an individual's original nature, how can we devise a treatment that might help them return to that state? With this aim in mind, I presented a detailed theory of 24 constitutional types in my previous book, along with the methods to determine and confirm this step in diagnosis. With several more years of clinical experience, I've decided that four of these constitutional types are null sets, that is, they have no members. I'd wager that most acupuncturists could make an accurate guess at the controversial types: they are constitutions whose primary tendency is either excess or deficiency of one of the systems associated with Ministerial Fire (xiang huo 相火),[3] being variously referred to as Heart Governor, Pericardium, Circulation-Sex, Ming Men,

2 "That which is tranquil from our birth is our heavenly nature. Stirring only after being stimulated, our nature is harmed" (Major *et al.* 2010, p.53).

3 By Ministerial Fire in this context, I am referring specifically to the functions commonly referred to in English as Pericardium and Triple Heater. I use the term Imperial Fire to refer to the functions referred to in English as Heart and Small Intestine. The term Ministerial Fire (xiang huo 相火) has other usages in Chinese medicine, and often refers to purely pathological conditions. In a posting (08/07/16) on the Facebook group Scholars of Chinese Medicine, Leo Lok clarified this confusing situation thus: "Zhudanxi very clearly disagrees with Lidongyuan in his writing the 'Treatise of Ministerial Fire' 相火論. To Zhu, in addition to the pathological state, there is a 'good' (physiologic) side to the Ministerial Fire, which is essential for the normal functioning of human physiology." I am extending the argument of Zhu by restricting the meaning of Ministerial Fire to only these normal functions of human physiology. This restricted definition only applies to this present treatise.

Heart Wrapping Network, Triple Heater, Triple Warmer, and Sanjiao, among other proposed names.

There is a simple reason why I began to suspect the need to delete these constitutions from the list of possibilities. In KCA, which contributed substantially to my earliest and ongoing training in acupuncture, the two meridians associated with Ministerial Fire are treated entirely differently from any of the other meridians. Kuon Dowon, who developed KCA, used one of the Ministerial Fire meridians (along with the meridian of their constitutional type) to treat cases of what he called neuro-psychological problems (among other indications).[4] He treated all the constitutional meridians with variations of the classical four-needle technique, but he treated the Ministerial Fire meridians with only two needles. Also, all of the non-constitutional meridians played fixed constellational roles related to the type of pathology present, so that the Spleen meridian could be treated for inflammatory conditions associated with the Fǔ Organ systems (gastritis, for instance) in one constitution (Liver Excess, for example), and alternatively chosen for treatment of inflammatory conditions of the Zang Organ systems (hepatitis, for instance) in another constitution (Kidney Deficiency, for example).[5] Only the Ministerial Fire meridians remained outside

4 Kuon used either Ministerial Fire meridians or Imperial Fire meridians to treat neuro-psychological problems depending on the individual's constitution. I believe this approach needed correction, limiting these treatments to Ministerial Fire in all constitutions, a proposal that was discussed in *The Compleat Acupuncturist.*

5 In Kuon's methodology, each individual has a four-needle combination of acupuncture points that is used to treat most problems of anyone having that constitution, called the basic or root formula. In addition, Kuon used other four-needle combinations of acupuncture points, focused on non-constitutional meridians, to focus the treatment on the specific pathology present, these other point combinations being called auxiliary formulae. The first of the auxiliary formulae that Kuon reported was the neuro-psychiatric one, alluded to in his initial 1965 publication. It consisted only of two acupuncture points, whereas all the subsequent auxiliary formulae contained four acupuncture points.

this constellational framework, treating the same pathological conditions regardless of the constitution. For this reason I came to the realization that KCA excepted constellational thinking (as I described it in Chapter 6 on the *Nan Jing*) from being applicable to the "Ministerial Fire" meridians. The logical consequence that proposition leads to is that in KCA there would be no Ministerial Fire types.[6]

It is interesting to think about the implications of Kuon's choice of neuro-psychological problems as being in the realm of Ministerial Fire. An easy association can be made between "neuro" and the jīng (essence 精), which is the basis of the brain and spinal cord ("marrow" 髓) in Chinese medicine, as well as an association of "psyche" and the *shén* (spirit 神) in Chinese medicine. Jīng and shén are at the less tangible end of the spectrum of the constituents of the human organism (being described as either non-material, or extremely subtle) in Chinese medicine. I discussed earlier the idea that being evolves from non-being in Chinese philosophy, and I have come to believe that Ministerial Fire plays a role in this aspect of creation. If my supposition is correct, it would explain why there are no constitutions based on Ministerial Fire, as inherent imbalances in the mechanism playing a role in the process of incarnation are probably incompatible with survival. The *jīng* is closely associated with the source qì (yuán qì 原氣) that is inherited from one's parents. The classics state that one of the functions of the Sanjiao is to distribute this source qì to the source points of all the principal meridians. Although most later texts refer to the yin meridian of Ministerial Fire by other

6 Honma Shohaku, one of the founding leaders of the Japanese Meridian Therapy style of practice, came to the same conclusion as I have, that is, that there are only 20 constitutional types, consisting of primary excesses or deficiencies of the principal meridians associated with the Five Elements, and in that case the Fire Element was represented by the Heart and Small Intestine meridians. His work has not been translated into English as far as I know, but he published many articles in the journal *Ido No Nippon* (for example, Honma 1949).

names, I think it is significant that the *Mai Jing* initially called it mìng mén 命門, or Gate of Life. Both of these traditional teachings support my contention that Ministerial Fire plays a role in the movement from pre-Heaven to post-Heaven, otherwise known as the movement from non-being to being, and acting as an intermediary between the source qì (yuán qì 原氣) and the qì of the zàng fǔ. My thoughts on this topic are illustrated in Figure A.2.

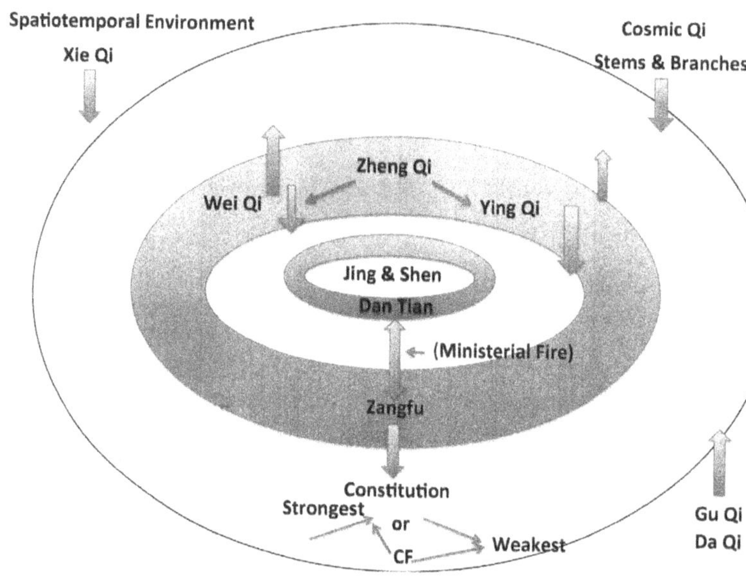

Figure A.2 A model of human organization
Source: Peter Eckman

A few words about the terminology in Figure A.2 are in order. The center of the human organism is often conceptualized as the dān tián (cinnabar field 丹田), which is often the place of concentration in meditation for the transmutation of jīng, qì, and shén traditionally located approximately two inches below the navel, in the abdomen. This spot is equivalent to the hara of Japanese teachings, being the site where the original ki (qì) is stored. The original or source qì needs to be distributed to the zàng fǔ and their principal meridians, and this function is the responsibility of the Sanjiao. Exactly what role mìng mén plays is unclear to me, but it would appear to complement the Sanjiao in distributing the vital force and individual nature from the unmanifest state of wú jí in the dān tián to the source points of the zàng fǔ in the manifest state of tài jí in the material body. The zàng fǔ and their meridians circulate zhèng qì 正氣 in the two forms (róng 榮 and wèi 衛 or yíng 營 and wèi 衛) discussed in the *Nan Jing*. The functioning of the normal (zhèng) qì can be disturbed by pathogenic factors (xié qì 邪氣) arriving from the exterior or interior, or even from improper lifestyle, such as diet. Actually, the influences (qì) from exterior, interior, and "neither" can be either pathogenic (xié) or normal (zhèng), depending on their appropriateness. Thus breath (dà qì 大氣), food (gǔ qì 穀氣), and emotional sources of nurturance contribute to healthy zhèng qì. As Simonov has posited, the cosmic qì generated by the interaction of the sun and earth are also supportive of healthy zhèng qì, and broaden the concept of dà qì to more than the air we breathe, or its oxygen content. Once the zàng fǔ have received their qì from its source in the dān tián, each individual expresses its constitutional typology according to which of the Organ systems is inherently prone to hyperfunctioning or hypofunctioning, depending only on their original qi supplied by Ministerial Fire from the source. This model, although a personal interpretation, is the best way I have found to integrate the teachings of the classics with their subsequent interpretation through the various styles of acupuncture espoused by Kuon, Simonov, and Worsley, among my other teachers.

If there are no Ministerial Fire constitutional types, how did my patients described as having that diagnosis benefit from the acupuncture treatments I described in *The Compleat Acupuncturist*? I recall hearing Worsley state that almost everyone can benefit from treatment of the Ministerial Fire meridians, and considering the role they play in supplying source qi to all the principal meridians, it is not an unreasonable observation. The cases I presented as having Ministerial Fire constitutions were all treated by Five Element protocols, rather than the four-needle technique of KCA, so the benefits they experienced from treatment can be explained without recourse to keeping a Ministerial Fire constitutional typology.

There is another part in the conceptualization in Chinese medicine, of how one's original nature, imparted at conception, is transformed from its unmanifested (wú jí) state into the incarnated human organism. I mentioned the embryological role of the extraordinary vessels in my discussion of the *Mai Jing*, but I'd like to emphasize that the creation of each individual being is not merely something that happens only at a specific time (the inception of life), but is constantly recreated every moment of that individual's life. As living organisms we are in a constant state of flux, losing cells, chemicals, and energy, but also replacing them anew all the time. Thus, our mechanisms of creation must also play an ongoing role in the maintenance of life. While this understanding is not explicitly described in relation to the extraordinary vessels in the classics (to my knowledge), I find that it provides a fuller ability to employ these vessels in acupuncture treatment than the more common explanation of them as simply "overflow reservoirs" to contain pathological (xié) qì that has overwhelmed the capacity of the principal meridians and their Organ systems to contain it. When a new human being starts life as a single cell, it is imperative that its future development can only proceed if it can maintain its internal orientation in space. It would certainly be tragic if our body parts developed in random places and with random orientations. Various Japanese and Korean styles of acupuncture emphasize the primary role of the extraordinary vessels in providing and maintaining this guiding organizational framework. Figure A.3 illustrates several of the implications of this interpretation of the functions of the extraordinary vessels. The terms first and second ancestry are adopted from the teachings of Jeffery Yuen, an inheritor of Chinese Daoist practices, including acupuncture. The Fu Xi and Wen Wang orders refer to arrangements of the trigrams of the *Yi Jing*, reminding me of why I chose this text for consideration in Chapter 1.[7]

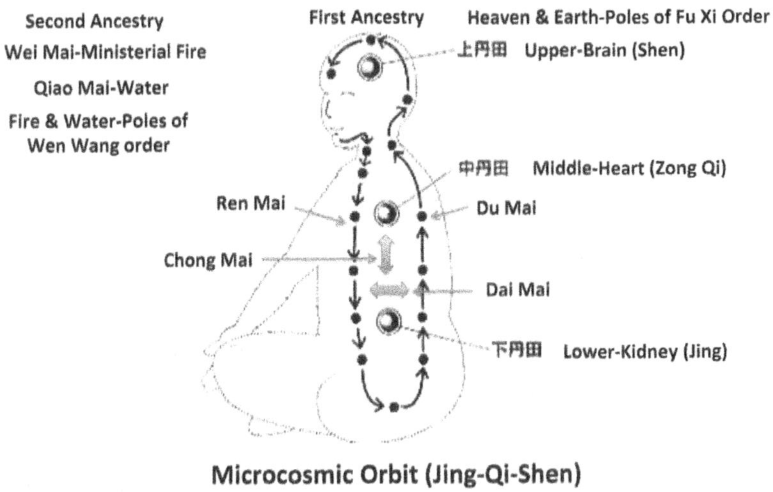

Figure A.3 Dan Tian and the extraordinary vessels
Source: Peter Eckman

When speaking of dān tián, the denotation refers to the location in the lower abdomen, unless specified otherwise, but an expanded version recognizes three dān tián, which makes it easier to visualize the Daoist teachings regarding the transmutation of jīng into qì and qì into shén, a process that reflects the spiritual path of Daoist adepts. The lower dān tián is the abode of the Kidneys, which are responsible for storing the jīng, but is also the site of mìng mén, which provides the Fire that enables this transmutation. The

7 The *Dao Zang*, a compendium of Daoist writings, contains many interpretations of Chinese medical thought, including material on the extraordinary vessels, which would otherwise be maintained only by oral transmission.

middle dān tián is the abode of dàn zhōng 膻中, which gathers our ancestral energy (zōng qì 宗氣), providing a connection to our lineage, as its main Organ systems of Heart and Lungs transmute gǔ qì, dà qì, and yuán qì into our individual zhèng qì, so that we can maintain our identity as individuals, but also as members of a familial lineage. Finally, the upper dān tián, where our brain is located, allows for the transformation of zhèng qì into shén, consciousness, or the light of spiritual awareness. The extraordinary vessels of the first ancestry (Du, Ren, Chong, and Dai) can be seen as establishing a three-dimensional grid of front vs. back, upper vs. lower, and interior vs. exterior. Ren mai and Du mai form what is called the microcosmic circulation, from the perineum to the crown and back again. Microcosmically it resembles the placement of Heaven and Earth in the Fu Xi order of the trigrams, at the top and bottom positions. The second ancestry consists of the Qiao mai and the Wei mai, whose opening points are on Water Element and Fire Element meridians respectively. Water and Fire trigrams form the orienting axis at the bottom and top of the Wen Wang order, often referred to as the Post-Heaven order, as distinguished from the Pre-Heaven order of the First Ancestry. This congruence of terminology Pre/First and Post/Second is a reminder that there is a logical coherency to the various theoretical constructs in Chinese medicine. Once again, Water (resonating with jīng) and Fire (resonating with shén) are seen to be operative in the creation and recreation of life in each individual.

A final correction, more of an adjustment really, of a topic presented in my previous book, is begging to be included here. In Chapter 7 on the *Mai Jing*, I alluded to the different finger positions for palpating the "yin" and "yang" pulses.[8] Previously I had

8 The yang pulse positions are those I have been describing for cùn, guān, and chǐ, with guān at the crest of the styloid process. The yin pulse positions are about one half cùn proximal, with the crest of the styloid process between the examiner's index and middle fingers. See *The Compleat Acupuncturist* for a detailed presentation of the theory of yin and yang pulse positions.

described these positions as providing information about the yin and yang status of the correlated Element respectively (e.g., the left cùn yang position resonates with the Heart and Small Intestine yang, while the left cùn yin position resonates with the Heart and Small Intestine yin). Radha Thambirajah's (2010) book on the Five Elements points out that, for example, the Heart yang is supplied by the Small Intestine, and the Small Intestine Yin is supplied by the Heart. On the basis of her teachings I have found that a simpler interpretation of the pulses felt at the yin and yang positions is accurate: the yang pulse position reflects the Fu Organ and meridian, while the yin pulse position reflects the Zang Organ and meridian. In a personal communication, Ross Rosen informed me that certain Tibetan methods of pulse diagnosis similarly differentiate the first and second half of the pulse wave analogously to what I have called the yang and yin pulse positions.

The reason I feel compelled to include this refinement here is that I didn't go into much detail about the correlations of the five depths of the pulse with the Five Elements as presented in *Nan Jing* chapter 5, as this topic was addressed in my previous book. Using the simplification suggested by Thambirajah's teachings, I find it is much easier to arrive at an accurate conditional diagnosis simply from attending to the pulse depth at cùn, guān, and chǐ at both the yang and yin locations. Appearing in the final two chapters of this treatise, I would like to emphasize how helpful the *Nan Jing* and *Mai Jing* are in arriving at a conditional and a constitutional diagnosis respectively. Other methods that I have described previously should not be ignored, but these two texts are, for me, the epitome of classical pulse diagnosis, and remain relevant more than two thousand years after they were written by astute observers, who were among China's earliest scientists.

In closing, I find myself thinking about the statue that prodded me to begin this treatise. Another statue is begging me to let it serve as the ending. Together, these works of art remind me that human nature has oft been perceived as deeply in the West as in the East. In my mind's eye, I can see William Shakespeare and Zhuāng Zǐ laughing together at what we might find at the Bottom of it all (Figure A.4), "but thereby hangs a tale."[9]

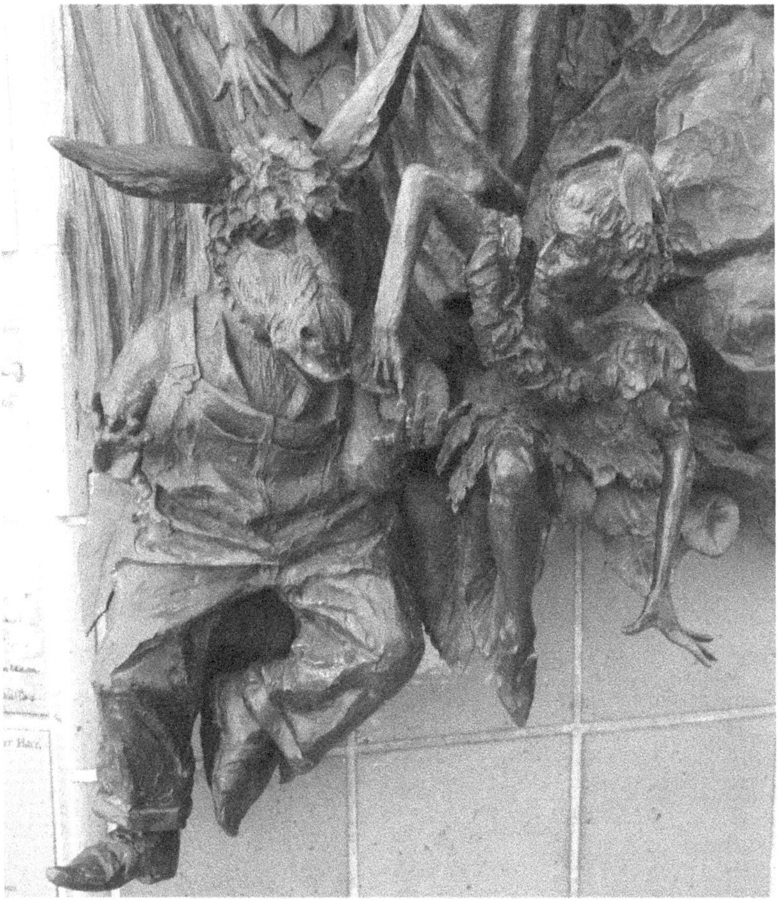

Figure A.4 Bottom and his muse; at the end of the donkey's tail
Source: Marina Chentsova Eckman

9 This expression, embodying the pun on *tail* and *tale*, was used by Shakespeare in at least four of his plays and presumably was well known before that.

REFERENCES

Blakney, R.B. (1980) *The Sayings of Lao Zi: A New Translation of the Tao Te Ching.* Taipei: Confucius Publishing House.

Buck, C. (2015) *Acupuncture and Chinese Medicine.* London: Singing Dragon.

Connelly, D. (1979) *Traditional Acupuncture: The Law Of The Five Elements.* Columbia, MD: Traditional Acupuncture Institute.

Eckman, P. (1983) *Closing the Circle: Lectures on the Unity of Traditional Oriental Medicine.* Fairfax, CA: Shen Foundation.

Eckman, P. (1988) *The Book of Changes in Traditional Oriental Medicine.* Columbia, MD: Traditional Acupuncture Institute.

Eckman, P. (2007) *In the Footsteps of the Yellow Emperor: Tracing the History of Traditional Acupuncture* (2nd Edition). San Francisco: Long River Press.

Eckman, P. (2014) *The Compleat Acupuncturist.* London: Singing Dragon.

Eckman, P. (2015) "Precision in finger placement for pulse diagnosis." *Journal of Chinese Medicine (UK) 109*, 49–55.

Ellis, A., Wiseman, N., and Boss, K. (1989) *Grasping the Wind.* Brookline, MA: Paradigm Publications.

Hammer, L. (2001) *Chinese Pulse Diagnosis: A Contemporary Approach.* Seattle: Eastland Press.

Hammer, L., and Bilton, K. (2012) *Handbook of Contemporary Pulse Diagnosis.* Seattle: Eastland Press.

Honma, S. (1949) *Keiraku Chiryo Kowa (Discourse on Meridian Therapy).* Yokosuka: Ido No Nippon. (In Japanese.)

Kaptchuk, T. (2000) *The Web that has no Weaver.* New York: Contemporary Books.

Kespi, J. (2012) *Acupuncture: From Symbol to Clinical Practice.* Seattle: Eastland Press.

Lavier, J. (1966) *Histoire, doctrine et pratique de l'acupuncture chinoise.* Paris: Tchou.

Le Blanc, C. (1985) *Huai-Nan Zi, Philosophical Synthesis in Early Han Thought: The Idea of Resonance (Kan Ying) With a Translation and Analysis of Chapter Six.* Hong Kong: Hong Kong University Press.

Lee Je-ma (1966) *Longevity and Life Preservation in Oriental Medicine.* Seoul: Kyung Hee University Press.

Major, J.S., Queen, S.A., Meyer, A.S., and Roth, H.D. (trans. and eds) (2010) *The Huainanzi; A Guide to the Theory and Practice of Government in Early Han China.* New York: Columbia University Press.

Mathews, R.H. (1979) *Mathews' Chinese–English Dictionary.* Cambridge, MA: Harvard University Press.

Needham, J. (1956) *Science and Civilization in China, Vol. 2.* Cambridge: Cambridge University Press.

O'Connor, J., and Bensky, D. (trans.) (1981) *Acupuncture, A Comprehensive Text.* Shanghai College of Traditional Medicine. Chicago: Eastland Press.

Omura, Y. (1982) *Acupuncture Medicine.* Tokyo: Japan Publications.

Porkert, M. (1995) *Classical Acupuncture: The Standard Textbook.* USA: Phainon.

Rosenberg, Z. (2013) "An interview with Paul Unschuld." *Journal of Chinese Medicine (UK) 103*, 1–8.

Scrimgeour, A. (2011) *What is the Relationship between the Yi Jing (The Classic of Change) and Chinese Medicine?* Bac. Dissertation. Reading: College of Integrated Chinese Medicine.

Thambirajah, R. (2010) *Energetics in Acupuncture.* Edinburgh: Churchill Livingstone.

Unschuld, P. (trans.) (1986) *Nan Jing.* Berkeley, CA: University of California Press.

Unschuld, P. (trans.) (2016) *Huang Di Nei Jing Ling Shu.* Oakland, CA: University of California Press.

Unschuld, P., and Tessenow, H. (trans.) (2011) *Huang Di Nei Jing Su Wen.* Berkeley, CA: University of California Press.

Van Meter, S. (2007) *Jingei Pulse Diagnosis.* Portland, OR: Working Class Acupuncture.

Wang Shu-he (1997) *The Pulse Classic: A Translation of the Mai Jing.* Trans. Yang Shou-zhong. Boulder, CO: Blue Poppy Press, 1997.

Watson, B. (trans.) (1964) *Chuang Tzu.* New York: Columbia University Press.

Wieger, L. (1965) *Chinese Characters.* New York: Dover Publications.

Wilcox, L. (2016) *Medicine and* The Changes *have the Same Source: The Relationship of Yì Jīng and Medicine.* Available at www.medicinalroots magazine.com/uploads/6/9/2/2/692250/medicinalrootsmagazine_fall16.pdf, accessed on 19 December 2016.

Wilhelm, R., and Baynes, C. (trans.) (1977) *The I Ching or Book of Changes.* Princeton, NJ: Princeton University Press.

Worsley, J. (1982) *Talking about Acupuncture in New York.* Royal Leamington Spa: The College of Traditional Chinese Acupuncture.

Wu, J. (trans.) (1991) *Yi Jing.* Washington, D.C.: The Taoist Center.

Yang, S. (trans.) (1997) *The Pulse Classic: A Translation of the Mai Jing.* Boulder, CO: Blue Poppy Press.